> *PRAISE FOR PETER PARK*

"Peter's been my trainer, workout partner, and friend since I was 12. No matter where I am in the world we talk almost every day. I would not be where I am now if it wasn't for Peter, no doubt."

—LAKEY PETERSON, professional surfer

"I have a tremendous amount of respect for Peter as a trainer, and I'm proud to call him my friend. He's developed incredible coaching wisdom through years of experience training clients and putting himself through rigorous workouts, and that wisdom generates results, plain and simple."

—BEN BRUNO, strength and fitness trainer

"For me Peter has been all things: fitness trainer, rehab coach, mentor, and trusted friend. He comes to many of my races, to the hospital after crashes, and is on the phone with me when I have questions or doubts. Except for me, no one is more committed to my success than Peter."

—KEN ROCZEN, Motorcross and Supercross champion

"I'm in the best shape of my life thanks to Peter."

—CHRIS SILBERMANN, President, ICM Partners

REBOUND

RE BOUND

> **REGAIN STRENGTH**

> **MOVE EFFORTLESSLY**

> **LIVE WITHOUT LIMITS**

AT ANY AGE

PETER PARK, JESSE LOPEZ LOW, JUSSI LOMAKKA AND WITH *JEFF KING*

Da Capo
LIFE
LONG

PERSEUS BOOKS | HACHETTE BOOK GROUP

Copyright © 2018 by Peter Park, Jesse Lopez Low, and Jussi Lomakka
Photographs © 2018 by Erin Feinblatt

Da Capo Press
Hachette Book Group
1290 Avenue of the Americas, New York, NY 10104
dacapopress.com
@DaCapoPR

Printed in the United States of America

First Edition: January 2018

Published by Da Capo Press, an imprint of Perseus Books, LLC, a subsidiary of Hachette Book Group, Inc. The Da Capo Press name and logo is a trademark of the Hachette Book Group.

The Hachette Speakers Bureau provides a wide range of authors for speaking events. To findout more, go to www.hachettespeakersbureau.com or call (866) 376-6591.

The publisher is not responsible for websites (or their content) that are not owned by the publisher.

Print book interior design by Tabitha Lahr.

Library of Congress Cataloging-in-Publication Data has been applied for.
ISBNs: 978-0-7382-1949-3 (paperback), ISBN: 978-0-7382-1950-9 (e-book)
LSC-C

10 9 8 7 6 5 4 3 2 1

DEDICATIONS

> PETER PARK

For my wife Kelly, whose unconditional love and support is the sole reason I am where I am today. And for my sons Hayden and Carter. Life did not make sense until I had you. You both inspire me more than you will ever know.

> JESSE LOPEZ LOW

For my parents, for their incredible support during the journey.
And Dr. Daniel Kalish, for bringing me back.

> JUSSI LOMAKKA

This book is gratefully dedicated to my family.

> JEFF KING

For Kathi King

CONTENTS

FOREWORD > BY PETER PARK

WHEN JOHN MURPHY CALLED ME a few years ago for training advice he had no idea he was about to become a guinea pig for this book. Neither did Mike Kelley or Chip Blankenhorn. Let me explain. Back in 2013 I coauthored *Foundation: Redefine Your Core, Conquer Back Pain, and Move with Confidence* with Dr. Eric Goodman. The book shared the training method we created to help people overcome back pain and move better. Developing Foundation Training had a big impact on the way I train my clients, whether they be young moms looking to get fit again, pro athletes trying to increase their performance, or the vast majority of people I train who used to "just do it"—just kill it on the bike or slopes—but weren't getting it done anymore. Although I've helped a lot of women and men Rebound during my thirty years as a fitness and strength coach, I wanted a specific test group for this book so I could pinpoint how long a successful Rebound takes. I defined success as losing excess weight, overcoming injury, and being able to return to full, out-of-gym activities like tennis, running, playing hoops, or planting a vegetable garden. So John Murphy's call couldn't have been better timed—and he couldn't have fit the Rebound bill more perfectly.

Like most of us, John had played high school sports, but later raced triathlons, even did a couple of Ironman races. But after many years in a high-stress desk job without time for exercise, John had gained a few pounds, had undergone surgery on both of his knees and both of his shoulders, and suffered from back pain. John's biggest weakness was his strength: He's a cardio guy and never really lifted weights, which was why he was so vulnerable to injury. He needed to get strong to overcome his aches and pains—and to prevent further issues. I agreed to take John on if he could find a few other guys looking to get back in shape.

John's first call went to Mike Kelley—perfect because I'd known Mike since high school. Back then Mike really used to get after it on the basketball and beach volleyball courts. After school Mike started his own construction company, so he was always active, he never let himself get out of shape, but he'd had back, knee, and shoulder surgeries, had gained a few pounds, and wasn't getting after it much anymore. Mike's Achilles' heel was cardio: He hated it, especially the "boring-as-sh--!" cardio machines like the stationary bike, the Concept 2 Ski-erg, and the Versa Climber. Perfect! I'd have to convert him. Mike became my second guinea pig.

The next call went out to Chip Blankenhorn, a former Stanford water polo player (go Cardinals!). Nowadays Chip works as an environmental consultant. At six-foot-three and 250 pounds, Chip was one big dude—too big, he agreed. And Chip is strong but had what I call "pool strength," which isn't very functional in the real world. Humans don't walk around breast stroking or flutter kicking in a weightless environment; under gravity's spell we must hinge or bend, squat and lunge—we walk and we run. Chip couldn't do any of those things well because over the years his movement patterns had deteriorated and he'd lost mobility. So poor movement became Chip's greatest weakness. He became guinea pig number three.

The first four weeks went like this: I convinced John, Chip, and Mike to change their high-carb, sugar-laden diets to one lower in carbs, naturally rich in (or cooked in) healthy fats, a moderate amount of protein, and an abundance of vegetables. Then we went to work on retraining their faulty movement patterns (which really challenged Chip) by practicing Foundation movements paired with some low-intensity cardio to rebuild their fitness base. And to get back their mobility, I taught them active-passive stretching and self-myofacial massage—foam rolling and smashing—to relieve their tight tissue.

After four weeks, when they were moving pretty well, they took the next step, loading those same movement patterns with weight (strength training, tough on poor John) followed by sessions of high-intensity interval cardio (Mike really struggled here). That's when their rebounding really took off. And over the course of six months they'd all lost the weight they needed to; they were strong, cardio-fit, looked great; and they were ready for the real world of tennis, golf, skiing—pretty much anything they wanted to do, without restrictions. So I had the answer to what might be your first of many questions: *How long will it take me to Rebound? Six months to build a solid foundation of fitness.*

Quick epilogue to my guinea pigs' story. After their six-month program was over, John, Mike, and Chip wanted to push themselves further, so they joined my Saturday morning workout group, two-hour-plus gruel-fests for me and some of my fittest friends like Steve Shlens, Lakey Peterson, and Ryan Leeton. After a couple of months of these Saturday workouts, Chip got so strong that I couldn't compete with him pushing the sled or racing on the SkiErg. John rebuilt his old cardio endurance to such a high level that he oftentimes beat me on the bike. And Mike? Mike's a beast, and he's back to getting after it all over again.

In honor of my guinea pigs John, Mike, and Chip, the last workouts in this book are called "Saturday Mornings." They're tough, but if that sounds daunting don't worry, I'll get you there. But, wait, hold on. Why should you trust me? You don't even know me, and the fitness and nutrition trades are ripe with hucksters and false prophets. Trust is an essential part of the trainer-client relationship.

Lucky for me, trust is also like a race—there to be won—and as you're about to learn, there's nothing I like more than a good race. Ready?

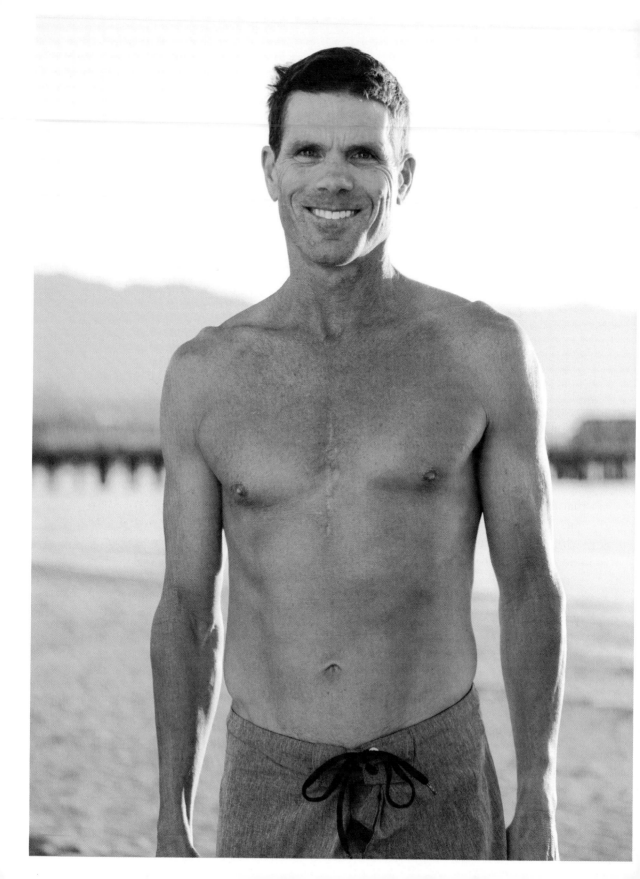

INTRODUCTION > BY PETER PARK

A LOT OF PEOPLE HAVE TOLD ME THAT I'm the most driven person they've ever met. That may sound like a compliment to you, but the reasons why I'm that way aren't exactly flattering.

I grew up in one of those huge families like you see in the movies, but ours was hardly a Hollywood fairy tale. I was the tenth of twelve kids, and my brothers, sisters, and I used to compete for everything—our parents' attention, food, sports, and even who'd ride shotgun in the old man's Buick. And if a poll had been taken among all us kids, I would've been voted "most competitive." I liked winning, sure, but I hated to lose a thousand times more.

But it wasn't just sibling rivalry that drove me to be so competitive. Genetics no doubt played a role. My dad had an obsessive nature too. He was a very successful engineer who built his own company from scratch, sold it, and retired at fifty—and then filled the void with drinking. Growing up watching him booze himself toward an early grave was hard on all of us. But my dad and I were so much alike, I was terrified I'd become an alcoholic too. For as long as I can remember, rather than deal with my fears and anxieties, I've run away from them, mainly by escaping through sports.

In junior high, when the other kids were hanging out at the beach or the mall, I was lifting weights at Santa Barbara Gym and Fitness, where I learned advanced strength-training techniques from some of the biggest, baddest power lifters in the country. If I wasn't weight training, I was probably on the volleyball courts at East Beach going against high school volleyball players like my then-mentor and idol, three-time Olympic gold medalist Karch Kiraly. Even though I was short in stature—or perhaps because of it—I outworked everybody, and in high school I made first-team, all-league volleyball all four years and earned a scholarship to play at the University of Hawaii.

After two years of playing collegiate volleyball I was itching for a new challenge, so I moved back home to Santa Barbara, where my dad was hitting the bottle even harder. So I hit the gym harder too, and in one year I added twenty-five pounds of muscle to my small frame. I was big, strong, and ripped, and I felt like I was in the greatest shape of my life. Then my younger sister, Jamie, who was attracting attention as a runner, challenged me to a 10k race. I don't remember why I accepted—she was fourteen, I was nineteen, in my prime, so maybe I figured there was no way she could beat me. Well, my baby sister crushed me. (Jamie later became the NCAA 10k champion.)

The loss cut right to the heart of my self-doubts. I had to find some way to prove I wasn't a failure, and the way my mind worked back then, the more punishing, the better. So on a whim I signed up for another race. But this race was different: instead of running a 10k (6.2 miles), I'd swim 2.4 miles, ride a bike 112 miles, and then finish by running 26.2 miles. My punishment for losing to my little sister was training for and competing in an Ironman triathlon.

There were problems right out of the gate. First, I didn't know anything about triathlons (is it bike first, then swim?) Also, I was a bad cyclist, an even worse swimmer, and you've already learned I wasn't a strong runner. But the biggest obstacle was time. The race was in just ten months, and I couldn't afford to hire someone to train me, so I was on my own. That's how I became a trainer: I took myself on as my first client.

I reached out to some triathletes I knew for training advice. Looking at my big muscles, they all said the same thing: "Stop lifting weights." I heard what they said, but I didn't listen. Sure, I hit the pool, road, and trails every day. But I also had this kind of crazy theory ("crazy" because no one I knew back then was doing it) that doing an Ironman—swimming, cycling, and running for nine-plus hours—certainly required cardio endurance but also endurance strength. If I was stronger than my competitors, that could give me a competitive edge. I sure as hell needed something! So I kept pumping iron. But I did make changes to my routine.

I had to slim down, so I switched from doing slow, isolating exercises (leg extensions, bench press, and bicep curls) that had made me big and bulky to circuits of compound, full-body movements (squats, lunges, and dead lifts), moving from one exercise to another at a quick tempo to build cardio and muscle endurance and strength all at once. Back at my old haunt, Santa Barbara Gym and Fitness, I got plenty of strange looks because no one was doing fast-tempo circuit training back then. I remember marveling that I could do a complete workout in the hour it took some guys to get through their six sets of bench presses. Then I'd fly out the door for a swim at Los Banos pool, cycle up Highway 154, and do a run up to the top of Gibraltar. My training days typically lasted six to eight hours. Pain, punishment, and escape became my life for the next ten months.

• • •

I arrived in Auckland, New Zealand, home of my first Ironman, weighing in at a lean and fit 150 pounds on race day—35 pounds lighter than when I started Ironman training. Nine hours and eight minutes later, I finished the race. It wasn't pretty, but I gutted it out and placed tenth overall. I turned some heads in the close-knit triathlon community: Who is this kid? Even so, I knew I could do better. I'd made a lot of mistakes in my training, and even before the race was over I was already planning what I'd do differently for the next one. And there would definitely be a next Ironman. I'd found my calling and the best way for me to escape.

But my racing career ran into another problem before it really got started. Ironman races don't pay much, even if you win (and I wasn't winning, not yet), and racing is not cheap: travel, doctor bills, equipment, millions of calories of food. Because I spent a lot of time in the gym anyway, I decided to hang up my own shingle and train other people. But how would I train folks who weren't looking to compete, who just wanted to get fit again? I'd learned from losing that 10k race to my sister that big muscles didn't translate to real fitness and had designed my new routine to give me a complete strength and cardio workout in about sixty minutes, easily done in a lunch hour. So I designed a program for those first clients based on my own fast-tempo circuit routine. And in so doing, I created a paradigm I'd use throughout my career: I became my clients' guinea pig. I'd write a workout for them, put myself through it first to hone and perfect it, and then it was their turn. Where I went they followed, over weeks, months, years. (Some of my first clients are still following me today.)

A few years into my racing career, my father crossed his own finish line. I was twenty-three. Even though his passing wasn't a complete surprise, I was so angry at the man. He'd given up, and that fractured our family. Unable to cope, I escaped deeper into my sport so I could deflect dealing with it, doing fifteen Ironman races over the next ten years. That's a lot of miles, and it's no coincidence I suffered every overuse injury in the book: tendonitis, chronic fatigue, torn calf, you name it. And on a training ride in Solvang I was hit by a car and suffered a broken wrist, leg, pelvis, separated shoulder, and a concussion. I suffered other injuries later on, which I'll talk about later.

But as physically painful and as deleterious to my career as those injuries were, I learned how to quickly recover from injury, and most of the time I came back stronger than before—and not to mention a little smarter. I finished my degree in kinesiology at UCLA, but to be honest, I learned more about the body's capabilities from recovering from my injuries than I did in school. And teaching myself how to get strong, flexible, and mobile again to speed up recovery made me more valuable to my clients trying to come back from their own injuries.

I used myself as a guinea pig when it came to nutrition too. When I started competing I was still existing on the junk food diet I grew up eating. But I learned pretty fast (dammit!) that Pop Tarts, burritos, and sugary chocolate milk don't power you very well through eight hours of swimming, running, and cycling. Once again I experimented on myself to find the best ways to refuel the human body. I tried every diet out there, from carbo-loading to strict veganism and vegetarianism, Atkins, Paleo, and even fasting. I put my body through the ringer, and although it took many years to get it right, I learned the best way to fuel my body for competition—and my clients' bodies for life. I'll talk about nutrition more specifically later on, but here's a hint: you've got to get back to eating real foods again, and that means a diet rich in good fats and tons of vegetables.

At the peak of my Ironman career I won the World's Toughest Triathlon three years in a row, and although my racing was going great, I'd developed a high-class problem: I had taken on a lot of clients, but I was running all over Santa Barbara to train them in different gyms. So finally I opened my own shop, Platinum Fitness, a gym hidden away in Montecito. I put together a team of trainers who, like me, were competitive athletes who needed to make cash to pay for their sport. Pretty soon my little gym turned into a performance-driven think tank and laboratory. Nobody outside of Santa Barbara—and for a while, even inside Santa Barbara—knew about us. We weren't rebels. We were BMX riders, beach volleyball players, and ultra marathon runners, experimenting and figuring things out together. Collaborating with these elite athletes helped advance my own training and my clients' workouts to a new level.

Starting my own business also meant I had new responsibilities. So did getting married and having two sons! I couldn't just take off to Hawaii, Tokyo, Sweden, or Germany to compete in Ironman races anymore. I had to grow up. (Just ask my wife, Kelly.) But I wasn't ready to retire, and having my own sons created new anxieties and new needs to escape. The compromise: I switched to doing mostly local ultra-marathons but started training even more. The result: for three years straight I won the Catalina fifty-miler and the Santa Barbara Nine Trails Ultra marathon.

I still mirrored my clients' gym workouts with my own—where I went they followed—and they moaned and groaned about our new levels of intensity. And my wife, Kelly, was doing some groaning herself. A former endurance athlete in her own right, a trainer, full-time recovery room nurse, mother of two, and, to be honest, the real force behind Platinum Fitness, Kelly understood what drove me and had always been sympathetic, but I was nearing forty, and she worried about the toll this level of training was taking on my body.

As usual, Kelly was right. I woke up one morning speaking gibberish, with the right side of my body numb. Kelly tried to get me to go to the ER. Instead, I went to train my first clients that morning, a group of doctors. They tried to get me to go to the ER. Instead, in complete denial, I cycled up and down one of the steepest hills in Santa Barbara ten times, trying to prove there was nothing really wrong with me. It didn't work. So, tail between my legs, I got myself to the ER for a proper diagnosis. After a battery of tests the doctors found a small hole in my heart called a PFO (patent foramen ovale) that was allowing small blood clots to enter my brain. I had suffered what they call a transient ischemic attack (TIA) and was in danger of having a more debilitating full-blown stroke. Two weeks later I had open heart surgery to repair the hole in my heart. After the surgery the doctor said I would heal completely, but instinctively I knew if I didn't back off, something else was going to give. For the sake of my family, maybe it was time to retire from competition.

Instead, as usual, I put off deciding about my racing future and spent my hiatus investing in my future as a trainer by learning more about the fitness industry. The first thing I did was make a pilgrimage to meet Russian kettlebell master Pavel Tsatsouline who embodied the qualities of a trainer that I respect most. Pavel is a terrific teacher and he practices what he preaches: the man's powerful and fit. He taught me the theory and discipline of kettlebell training, one of the most efficient ways to build strength. He liked my circuit training but advised me to simplify my workouts and focus on building strength. Pavel has become a good friend, we talk shop often, and he continues to be a big influence in my strength training, and by extension, he will be on yours too.

Over time I could feel myself getting stronger. I started testing myself doing weights and light cardio at Platinum Fitness. And then a once-in-a-lifetime opportunity came knocking that would change my life. A pro cyclist who himself had just retired from competition asked me to train him. I'd made a name for myself as an athlete in the small Ironman and ultra-marathon circles, but as a trainer I thought no one outside Santa Barbara had even heard of me. He wasn't looking for someone to just tell him what to do; he wanted a training partner to run and cycle up mountains with, do hardcore strength training alongside, someone who could push him every step of the way. That's why he chose me, because I was one of the few trainers who might be able to keep up with him. In fact, at the time this guy—Lance Armstrong—was the best endurance athlete in the world.

Okay, I know, and say what you will about Lance, but I've trained and trained with the best athletes in the world, and I can tell you unequivocally that Lance outworks them all. I've never seen anyone with his work ethic, his everyday persistence, and his willingness to push himself past his own limits. Over the coming months he would challenge me in ways I'd never faced before. So for me personally, to go up against Lance on the bike, on the trails, and in the gym—forget the money and what training him might do to further my career—as I said, this was the opportunity of a lifetime. The doctor gave me clearance (though not his blessing), and I went for it.

I didn't tell Lance that I was recovering from open heart surgery. I didn't want him to slack off, and I sure as hell didn't want his pity. Turned out Lance and I are kindred spirits, we're driven by many of the same demons, and our families became close friends.

Lance's training went so well that he decided to make a comeback and ride the Tour de France again. We trained together on the bike in Santa Barbara, Aspen, and Texas for several months before he left for Europe. And my own training was going so well that I was inspired to make a comeback too. But it never happened. Because when Lance took off he left behind a parting gift that would change my future.

Lance told some guys in LA about how I trained him (and by "guys" I mean heavy hitters in the entertainment and sports management businesses). They liked that I focused on getting fit and healthy, not absurdly ripped like those airbrushed, half-starved guys on magazine covers. Next thing I knew, I was training A-list actors, musicians, and other celebrities and making more money than I ever thought I would. I was getting asked to write for fitness magazines, sitting courtside at Laker games, and meeting a lot of connected people who knew more connected people. It was totally surreal!

Around that time I met Dr. Eric Goodman, a young surfer-chiropractor whose field of study focused on people suffering from lower back pain. The chief cause of back pain these days is our sedentary lifestyles—sitting on our asses all day—which takes a toll on our posture. It can also destroy our natural movement patterns: how we walk, run, bend over to pick up our keys. And as I'd seen with so many of my clients over the years, these faulty patterns cause pain and sometimes injury.

Eric wanted me to help him develop a program with the specific goal of helping people get out of pain without surgery or prescription drugs. We focused on retraining the posterior chain of muscles that run from the back of the legs up through the glutes and into the lower back, our true core and power center. We developed a handful of specific movements and were surprised how quickly and effectively they helped people who'd been living with back pain for years, or even decades. We gave it a name: Foundation Training, and published a book, *Foundation: Redefine Your Core, Conquer Back Pain, and Move with Confidence*. Eric is a medicine man, and his focus is helping people heal. I'm a performance guy, and I saw the potential Foundation Training could have to improve my clients' fitness level.

Back in LA I started training Casey Wasserman, one of the top sports agents anywhere, and his training went so well that he asked me to work with a few of his clients, many of them the best, highest paid athletes in the world. Most had worked with team trainers in college and the pros, so they could move pretty well, right? No. Most couldn't even do basic movements like squats or hinges. Why? A lot of them were never taught how to. But also, these pitchers, hitters, point guards, quarterbacks, and boxers had been doing sports-specific exercises that mimicked the same movements they did a hundred or a thousand times every day while practicing or playing their sport. It was all about performance narrowed down to a few, sports-specific exercises. To me that made no sense. They were digging grooves while playing their sport—faulty grooves a lot of the time—then going to the gym and digging them even deeper. I started all these top athletes the same way we'll get started in this book: unweighted Foundation movements until you're moving right. Only then do we add weight to the movement. It works for the pros, and it will work for you.

So what about my own racing career? I knew it was time to hang up my running shoes, but of all the challenges I've faced, from Ironman competitions to coping with my inner demons, retiring from competition was the hardest. Athletes are defined by our sport, but if we're not competing anymore, then who are we? My dad went through something similar. After he retired from running his company he had no answer for the question, "Who am I now?" And he fell into an alcohol-fueled depression. But when I retired that didn't happen to me.

I am still fueled by the complexities of growing up in a family with addiction. And I still may be the most driven guy you've ever met. But I've found ways to deal with my obsessive nature besides killing myself on the bike, in the water, and on the trails. Helping people heal helps me heal—and I'm eager to get you started. I hope you trust me now.

As a trainer, I have three primary points of emphasis: strength, flexibility, and mobility. My goal—both for myself and for my clients—is to balance these three pillars of fitness, ultimately resulting in pain-free activity and an uninhibited pursuit of life. Whether it's hiking, biking, running, swimming, or something as simple as playing with your kids jumping on a trampoline, I want you to be able to enjoy these activities and your body and to be able to fully explore all that you're capable of—without pain. For me this means pursuing my passions outdoors: snowboarding, surfing, wakeboarding (I like to go fast), and, of course, basketball. I feel extremely fortunate that I am able to do each of 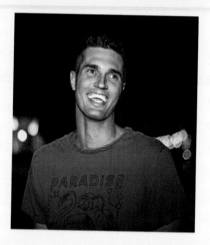 these activities—pain-free—because for a long time I wasn't able to.

During my freshman season playing basketball at UC Davis I began to develop chronic back pain in my lower back. As I'm sure you know, back pain makes it pretty difficult to do just about anything, let alone compete in Division 1 college basketball. To make matters worse, I contracted a rare autoimmune disorder. It seemed like I was always sick; I felt constantly exhausted and had very little energy for anything. And being a scholarship member of the basketball team, this was a big problem for me. My teammates could recover from a grueling practice or tough game in a matter of hours, but I needed days to recover. I knew something was wrong, so I went to every doctor and specialist I could find, but to no avail. Ultimately the disease forced me to quit before my senior year. It destroyed my ability to do what I loved most, and if you've ever had a pain or illness keep you from pursuing your passions, then you know exactly how this feels: terrible.

I realized that if I was ever going to get well, I'd have to take it upon myself to find answers. So after I graduated I started to travel, both domestically and abroad. I visited gyms, went on retreats, spoke with counselors, consulted chiropractors (for my back), and read every book I could that might potentially lead me to a resolution. I spent years soul searching to discover who I am and how to overcome my illnesses.

The first major breakthrough on my road toward recovery was discovering how nutrition could help me manage my autoimmune disorder. By cutting out gluten, grain, carbs, sugar, and alcohol, I felt better than I had in years. Then my second breakthrough occurred when I met Peter (Park) and Dr. Eric Goodman. They introduced me to their Foundation program, which helped me overcome my chronic back pain and had me feeling like my old self again.

Each of these discoveries made me hungry to learn more about the human body and how it's designed for optimal performance. So I packed up and moved to Santa Barbara to fully commit myself to my own health and well-being, becoming a personal trainer and Foundation instructor while working and learning directly from Peter. Combining what I learned from Peter, my own experiences with clients, and my study of other modalities and teachers, I was able to develop and refine those core principles of movement, training, and nutrition into a singular method. I call it TruMethod. I knew I was onto something important, something that needed to be shared, spread far and wide. People needed to know what I knew so they could break free from pain and enjoy their bodies to their maximum potential. So Peter and I spoke, and we came up with the idea that we should write a book together, chronicling our discoveries and independent journeys toward becoming our best selves. This is how *Rebound* was born.

JUSSI LOMAKKA

As a child in Finland I was captivated by sports, and after devoting many years to the practice of ice hockey, soccer, wrestling, and bandy I learned that to perfect training, you must understand anatomy and movement. My education started in Helsinki, Finland, at the Sports Massage and Rehabilitation Institute, followed by my specialized degree for joint manipulation, spine, myofascial, and trigger therapy from the TR Institute in Seinajoki, Finland. My education gave me a strong foundation and left me with a desire and passion to continue to learn and grow.

I have dedicated myself to a lifetime of service to others, which has resulted in work that has included traveling with the U2 360 Tour and Stars on Ice, several years with the San Francisco Ballet, and a thriving private practice in Malibu for over thirteen years in addition to working with numerous other professional athletes and celebrity clients.

Peter and I share many clients. He does the training; I keep them moving. It is a great relationship that I value very much.

Are you still unsure if this program is for you? Do you have more questions before you jump in? That's okay—I anticipate lots of questions as we go and will answer them all throughout the book. Let's tackle a few basic issues upfront so you can get moving.

QUESTION: What does the Rebound program look like?

ANSWER: There are five elements to the Rebound program: nutrition, cardio, movement, strength, and recovery (flexibility-tissue). In the coming chapters I go over each of them in detail so you'll know what to expect as you start training. When you actually start working out, you'll begin with four weeks of retraining your movement patterns in a chapter called Movement Practice. During those four weeks you'll get your body moving right again; begin low-level, base-building cardio exercise; and begin tweaking your eating habits. After those first four weeks you'll begin strength training and high-intensity interval training. The fifth element is recovery: stretching and deep myofascial massage designed to improve your mobility and suppleness of your tissue.

QUESTION: How often should I work out?

ANSWER: I expect that you'll dedicate yourself to training three times a week. Day One and Day Three are the same workout except for a tweak to cardio. Day Two is movement practice and low-intensity cardio to keep you on track. (Note: never strength train two days in a row.) I also recommend you take a weekend day and go on a long bike ride or hike to help further develop your base-building cardio fitness level.

QUESTION: You talk about spending a lot of time learning cues and how to move again. But I'm in decent shape and used to lift weights, so can I skip ahead and go straight to the workouts?

ANSWER: No, but thanks for asking. Trust me: first, you need to learn all the techniques to do the Rebound workouts correctly and safely. My method of training truly is different from what you're used to. And then you need to learn how to move well again and build a good cardio base, just like the pro athletes I train. That lays the foundation for the strength training. To use the old architect's metaphor, you wouldn't build a house on a shaky foundation. So don't build your fitness on unsteady ground.

QUESTION: I've never used kettlebells. Will that be a problem?

ANSWER: No problem at all. Most gyms have kettlebells now, and if you plan to work out at home, kettlebells are readily available, not too expensive, and you only need a few. As for the mechanics of using kettlebells, I spend a great deal of time teaching you the techniques and cues. It does take work, but I think you're going to love using kettlebells as much as I do—they are super-intuitive and the best and most efficient way to get strong again.

QUESTION: My shoulder, my knee, or my lower back hurts. Should I even do these workouts?

ANSWER: At the risk of sounding like a bad infomercial, if you have a serious injury like a torn rotator cuff or ACL, a groin tear or a slipped disc, or if you have a heart condition, see your doctor first. He or she might recommend physical therapy or testing before you begin your program. But if your shoulder or knee hurts from normal wear and tear, tendonitis, or osteoarthritis, and your lower back aches from sitting on your butt all day, the Rebound workout can actually help you overcome some—if not all—of your aches and pains. That is the heart and soul of this book.

QUESTION: I may be out of shape, but I'm not overweight. Do I still need to change the way I eat?

ANSWER: You don't have to do anything you don't want to. But I advise you to read the chapter on nutrition when you begin this program, because your body is going to have different nutritional needs. I'll show you how to fuel up for maximum performance and recovery.

> ACKNOWLEDGMENTS

PETER PARK: The foundation for this book started when I was a kid, so there's a million people who've contributed to its making in one way or another along the way.

I consider myself the luckiest man on the planet for having the best mentors anyone could luck into, like Don Johnson, Ed Snider, Casey Wasserman, and Irving Azoff. Maybe I was in search of a father figure. I found a bunch of them. Lance Armstrong showed me what a real work ethic looks like. Without him I wouldn't be where I am now.

All the coaches I have worked with and looked up to: Pavel Tsatsouline, Phil Maffetone, Ben Bruno, and especially the ones at my side at Platinum Fitness, who've pushed me—we are one big family.

My relationships with Eric Goodman and Tim Brown taught me more about how the body works than anything I've done in my career.

Barry Cappello has been a friend and mentor and has helped me in so many ways.

Jeff King, our writer, went a thousand times above and beyond the call of duty. I will miss our countless conversations and Saturdays together. Without you, this book would have never happened.

Jesse and Jussi, thanks for pushing me to become a better trainer and person. It was a fun journey.

Eric Feinblatt is a terrific photographer who understands how to translate what I do into photographs that are gems.

JESSE LOPEZ LOW: I want to thank Peter Park for the collaboration on this book and project, my clients for the opportunity to work with them, and my friends and family who have supported me throughout this journey.

JUSSI LOMAKKA: I must thank my wife, Julie, who is the true north in our family and whose morals we live by.

I also must thank my daughter, Emmi, who keeps teaching me how to be a better parent, person, and father.

Thanks to all my clients, mentors, and teachers with whom I have crossed paths along my own journey that began in northern Finland.

The Arctic Circle: the weather was so cold there that of course I found myself here in beautiful California.

And here in California is where I met Peter Park, whom I've grown to respect tremendously. Peter's the second-best trainer out there—though if there's someone better, I have not heard of them, so for now, Peter, when people ask, I'll say you're the best. Thanks for asking me to be a part of your book!

And last but not the least I am grateful to my parents, Reino Lomakka and Leila Lomakka, as well as my sister, Outi, who was truly an angel and a good artist in her own right. I know I'm right when I say that heaven got a heck of an artist up there.

What I learned from my family is to keep dreaming and working hard. I feel like life is nothing but a treasure hunt: you follow the clues from the universe, and you'll find the treasure at the end.

JEFF KING: I learned a ton from Peter Park during the writing of this book.

At ICM I'd like to thank Chris Silbermann, who has stuck by me and can deadlift more than me; Kristyn Keene, who is savvy and a true mentor; and Miranda King, my hero.

Closest to my heart, Duncan King. You've taught me more than you know.

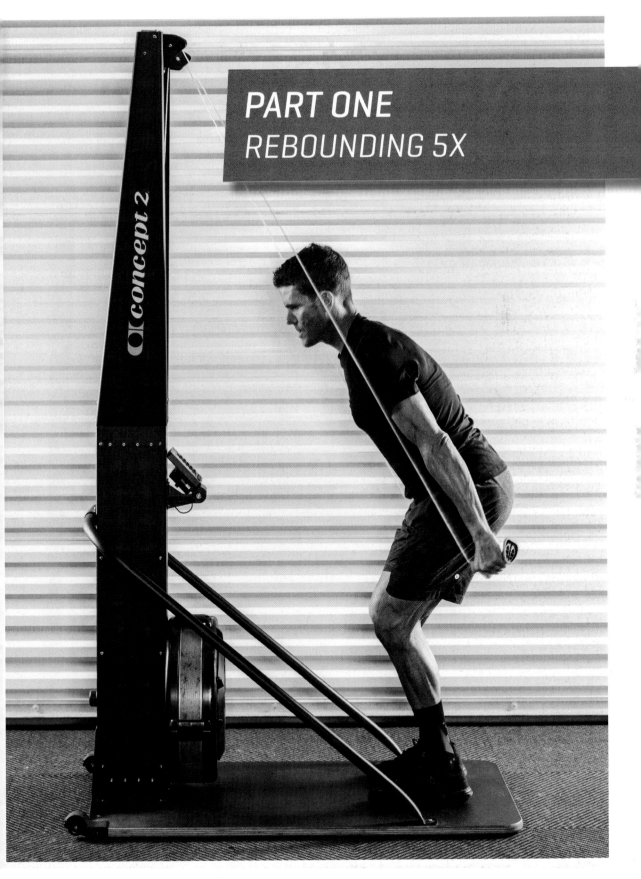

PART ONE
REBOUNDING 5X

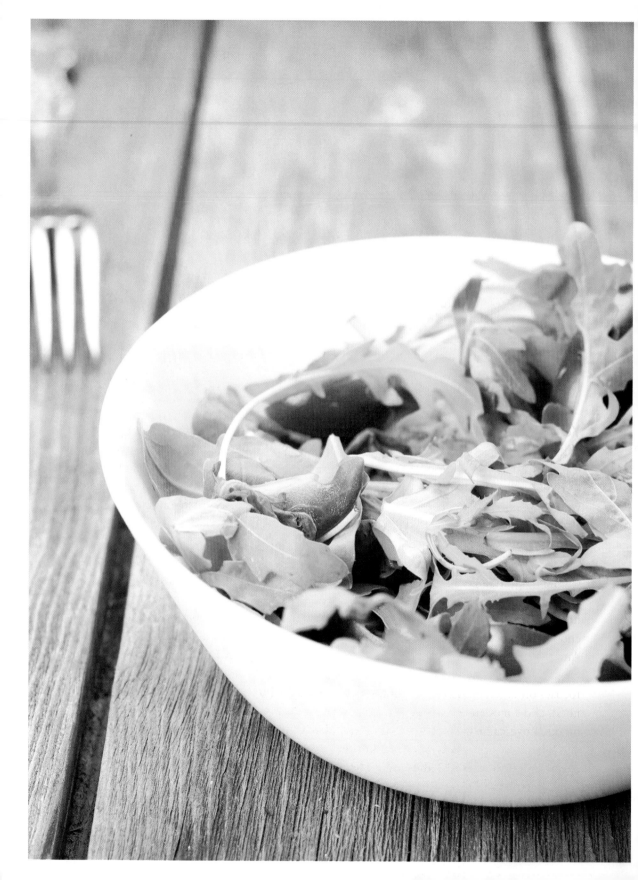

CHAPTER ONE: NUTRITION

YOU'VE LIVED A LOT OF LIFE, worn tread off your tires (but there's still plenty left!), you've celebrated successes, and punished yourself for your mistakes. But you've learned from them. And now you're on the road to rebounding, where you'll learn how to move well again and regain strength and cardiovascular fitness as well as get back your lost flexibility and supple tissue. To get there will require your persistence, patience, and hard work. But the most challenging part of the 5x program for you might be changing the way you eat.

Food's complicated. I've worked with people who have some serious eating disorders, terrible eating habits, and nasty food addictions. Some plan their days, weekends, and even vacations around where and what they're going to eat. (Sound familiar?) I'm not judging them. (Or you.) I get it: the other day I bought an expensive bar of dark chocolate, ate two bites, then tossed the rest in the trash for fear I'd eat the whole thing. And then I felt like an idiot for my lack of self-control. Not my finest moment, but that kind of thing doesn't happen to me so much anymore. By shifting my diet to one that focuses on vegetables, foods naturally rich in good healthy fats (like avocados, eggs, and nuts), and a moderate amount of protein while cutting down on sugar and carbohydrate intake, I overcame most of my food issues. Here's how it happened.

Like most other kids, I was cuckoo for Cocoa Puffs. Lays potato chips? No way I could eat just one. And I absolutely wanted to buy the world a Coke and keep it company. But when I first started training for Ironman races, I couldn't last 10 miles on the

GETTING BACK ON THE HORSE
By actor Don Johnson

While doing a horse stunt during the *Django Unchained* shoot I suffered a pretty serious injury, separating my pubis symphysis and tearing my abs in three places. It hurt like hell to move around, so I didn't much, and the pounds started creeping on. I switched to eating vegan, but damn if I didn't gain even more weight. My wife kept bugging me to go see this trainer, Peter Park, but I'd worked with a bunch of the so-called fitness gurus before. Well, turns out Peter's nothing like those guys. He's a uniquely intuitive, physiological miracle worker. First, he helped me get up and moving again. And he got me to change my diet to mostly healthy fats and to doing low-intensity cardio that burned that fat, so my input and output were talking to each other. Eventually I got super-fit again, my weight's now the same as it was in high school, and I'm stronger than I've been in my life, which is a good thing, because I have a lot of kids, and I'm working like crazy these days!

bike, let alone 110, eating and drinking those nutrient-deprived, chemically enhanced, sugar-rich, superfluous calories. So I had to make changes. But for many years that junk food I grew up eating still called my name, like drugs to an addict.

Of course that's no surprise. Like most drugs, these "foods" are created in laboratories precisely to *be* addictive (the sugary ones especially) because the people who sell them want us coming back for more. And more and more. So don't blame yourself for craving those salty chips or the sugary sodas and candy you've been eating all your life. Like other addictions, food dependency can be hard to overcome. But an important part of this journey you're on is saying, "Okay, but from now on…" The good news is that if you're willing to admit you have a problem, making these changes to the way you eat can help with your recovery.

As I mentioned in the Introduction, I experimented with every method of fueling myself for training and competition, and by the late 1980s I found what I thought was the best of them. And it came with a pedigree. The method was based on the research of Dr. Timothy Noakes, then the leading sports nutritionist in the world. Dr. Noakes advised his athletes to focus their diets on carbohydrates—or carbo-loading. This makes sense because carbohydrates convert to sugar in our bodies, and sugar is a quick and powerful source of energy. When we carbo-load, our bodies can store about four to five thousand carbohydrate/sugar calories, which is quite a lot of fuel in the tank (two days' worth for the average male).

But for an endurance athlete like me it wasn't enough. During training or racing an Ironman or ultra-marathon I'd burn six, seven, or eight thousand calories and have to deficit spend. How did I make up the deficit? When I felt my energy levels sagging—when my gas tank was running low—I'd wolf down a couple of energy gels. The glucose and fructose in the gels are designed to normalize blood sugar and delay the emptying of the glycogen tank. In other words, gels are pure octane and kicked me back in gear—well, until their fleeting energy burned off, I started running on fumes again, and then I'd have to throw down some more. During the average race I'd eat ten to fifteen gels just to make it to the finish line.

I was still riding the high-carb energy roller coaster when, in 1991, I met Dr. Philip Maffetone, an endurance sport coach and nutritionist. He said we were getting the diet thing all wrong, especially endurance athletes like me who carbo-loaded. Dr. Maffetone believed ultra-distance athletes like me should be using fat as our primary fuel source, not carbohydrates and sugar, because fat burning is more efficient: the human body stores about five times as many fat calories as it does sugar and protein calories. In other words, our fat fuel tanks are way bigger, which means we don't have to refuel as often. He also believed that eating good fats was flat-out healthier than a high-carb diet, and not just for athletes. Refined carbohydrates can impair fat oxidation rates, or the conversion of stored body fat into aerobic energy, which causes weight gain, and too many carbs and sugar can also cause inflammation, diabetes, and maybe even cancer.

Dr. Maffetone informed me that if I ate foods high in good fats as fuel, my energy levels would stabilize, I wouldn't have those sugar highs and lows during training and races anymore, and my performance would likely increase. Armed with his advice, I jumped right into eating a healthy-fats diet. Wait—no, I didn't. Athletes have a tendency to be superstitious, at least when they're winning, and I didn't want to fix what wasn't broken, so I kept on fueling myself with carbs.

And for a while carbs did the trick. I won the Catalina 50 Mile Ultra and the Nine Trails Ultra back-to-back in 1998 and 1999 while still carb fueling. But I was getting older, not recovering as quickly from my training as I used to, and, quite honestly, it was a pain in the ass to have to refuel so many times a day. Like our primal ancestors, it seemed like I was spending half my time hunting and gathering food. And I couldn't help thinking about what Dr. Maffetone said: our bodies can store twenty-five thousand calories of fat. That's enough stable energy to run four ultra-marathons without eating a bite of food! I couldn't resist any longer, so in late 1999 I decided to adapt to a healthy fats diet.

So what exactly is a good or healthy fats diet? I like to think of it this way. For its whole life up until that point, my body had primarily used its "carbohydrate tank" for energy. But now I needed to train it to tap into my vast fat stores. To do it I cut down on carbohydrates (no more than 100–150 grams per day) and ate mostly plant-based foods either raw, steamed, or cooked in healthy fats and a moderate amount of protein. For example, I started my day eating two eggs; a handful of spinach or kale cooked in a little olive, avocado, or coconut oil; avocado; a touch of cream in my coffee; and for carbs a small serving of sweet potatoes, quinoa or a handful of blueberries or raspberries (yes, berries have sugar but also antioxidants, and vitamins). These dense calories really stick with you, and I found that I didn't get hungry again for five, six, or even seven hours. I also noticed that I wasn't having the sugar-induced highs and crashes during training anymore, just like Dr. Maffetone projected. And once I became adapted to this new way of fueling myself, I started feeling more energetic and recovering from workouts more quickly.

(**NOTE:** When I did high-intensity interval workouts, I ate more carbs—150 to 200 grams a day—because high-intensity training taps into glycogen stores. You'll do the same when you start high-intensity interval training, adding foods like sweet potatoes, quinoa, and brown or white rice in small portions back into your diet. On sedentary or base-building days, however, you'll keep the carbs at bay. Much more on that later.)

On the day of the 2000 Catalina Ultra I was excited to see how I'd perform. During the race I fueled only with electrolyte replacement and a higher-fat, lower-sugar drink to power me through. Over the five hours and forty-five minutes it took me to finish, I never felt the highs and lows of that energy roller coaster I had encountered in the past. And I broke the course record by twenty minutes. My experiment of using fat as my primary fuel for racing was a rousing success!

But what's that got to do with you? You're just trying to break bad habits, lose a few pounds, and get healthier, not set ultra-marathon records. That's what two of my longtime clients, Barry Cappello and Ed Snider, barked back at me when I made them my nutrition guinea pigs. Both were highly successful guys in high-stress jobs. Both loved their sugary, nonfat, processed junk foods, but when they saw the success I had with shifting my diet, they gave it a try, eating a lot of green vegetables raw or cooked in healthy oils, visiting salad bars, eating more eggs and occasionally a couple of strips of bacon while keeping their carbs down. Right away they both dropped weight and continued losing over time, and both said they felt better overall, had more steady energy throughout their workday, and didn't have the gnawing hunger that used to plague them throughout the day. But maybe the most important upshot for them both—and the key to coping with food phobias, addictions, and stubbornness to make changes—is that Ed and Barry said changing their diet to eating real food, the same kind of foods our great grandparents ate back in the day, truly satisfied them and wiped away a lot of their cravings for and addictions to potato chips, muffins, donuts, fast food, and soft drinks.

Despite all of the evidence that changing their diets would help my clients lose weight, get leaner, feel better, and improve their athletic performance, I still had one reservation: from a health standpoint, was it fool's gold? What does eating a diet rich in healthy fats do to your HDL (good cholesterol), LDL (bad cholesterol), and triglycerides levels? I believed what Dr. Maffetone said, and the US government nutritional guidelines had just switched back to recommending eggs and other healthy fats, but doctors and governments have been known to be wrong. Just because I saw amazing outward results in myself and my clients, did that mean we were healthier on the inside too?

I'm a fanatic about getting frequent physical exams, since my engine logs a lot more miles than the average human's. And after I changed my diet, my HDL levels went up a lot (which is good), my LDL went down (again, a positive), and my triglycerides went down as well. The same thing happened with Ed and Barry. And after Don Johnson changed his diet, his doctor called me in disbelief because Don's triglycerides and bad cholesterol had dropped like a stone. "What did you do to him?" he asked.

My skepticism is long gone. Even Dr. Timothy Noakes, the sports nutritionist and one-time carbo-loading advocate I had originally consulted with pulled his own U-turn on carbo-loading in 2007 and began preaching the virtues of eating a healthy-fats, low-carb diet.

Okay, I know: cutting down on carbs and sugar sounds intimidating and even counterintuitive (eating more fat makes me lose weight?) But in fact it's really, really easy and cool because you're gaining a lot more than you're sacrificing. You get to fill your breakfasts, lunches, and dinners with great-tasting, honest, real food and let go of the overly processed, fake crap that's killing you bite-by-bite. The biggest challenge might be on base-building and no-exercise days when you should keep your carbohydrate intake to 100 to 150 grams a day or even lower.

I've given you a lot of information, and I recognize that making big changes to the way you eat is challenging. So I'm going to take a pause and answer some questions that many of my clients have asked me and you might be wondering about too.

QUESTION: I've tried every diet in the world and never had lasting success, and now you want me to go down that road and feel like a failure all over again? Seriously?

ANSWER: Eating a lot of fresh, tasty vegetables, a moderate amount of eggs, a touch of dairy, fish, steak, chicken, and even bacon isn't a diet; it's a return to eating the way people used to before the American diet got turned on its head. It's eating the way you should've been eating your whole life. You probably heard someone say you must fail to succeed? You've done enough failing. Time to put all that behind you and move on. *Seriously.*

QUESTION: I have a lot of food allergies and therefore restrictions, and my body doesn't tolerate lactose well. What would you recommend for me diet-wise?

ANSWER: Even with all your restrictions, eating good fats can work for you. It's always smart to check with your doctor or nutritionist before you start something new, but I've worked with a lot of people with similar food restrictions as you, and they had no problem making the change to a plant-based, healthy fats diet.

QUESTION: I cannot eat meat for humane reasons, and that's why I've never tried Paleo. Your diet sounds a lot like Paleo. So what should I do?

ANSWER: Paleo and fat adapting have some things in common. But the foundation of my nutrition plan is eating vegetables, so you should be fine. You just need to find alternative protein sources. Because you're a vegetarian, you probably already eat a lot of nuts, eggs, and dairy (if your conscious permits), quinoa, hummus, leafy greens, and other protein-rich foods. But you bring up a wider issue: no two people are alike, and one size does not fit all. Adapting to a healthy-fats diet for you might look different from someone else. For instance, are you the "all or nothing" type, like my client, Tina, an MD and marathon racer who was a big believer in carbo-loading? Once Tina researches a subject, considers its feasibility, and makes a conclusion, she's in and never looks back. Tina adopted a plant-based, healthy-fats diet and indeed never looked back. Are you the suspicious or more cautious type of person, like Mark, a talent manager in his late sixties whose years working in the music business with some of the world's top acts has taught him to question everything and everybody? Mark is suspicious of change, so he experimented, found foods he liked, rejected some parts of the plant-based, healthy-fats diet, and, over a few months, created his own version of a healthy-fats diet. Or you may have other challenges, like my guinea pig John Murphy, who has a compulsive nature and was eager to lose the twenty-five extra pounds he'd put on so was all in from day one. Typically John ate zero carbs for several weeks, but when faced with tight deadlines at work and a ton of stress, he gave in to his sugar cravings. I talked him back, and over time he adapted to a more conservative version of the diet and lost the twenty-five pounds. Tina, Mark, and John are all different people. Who are you? Discovering the answer over these next six months might teach you a lot about yourself.

QUESTION: I suppose this means you're going to ask me to cut sugar out of my diet, right? I love sugar—and sugar loves me. So if I have to stop eating sugar, forget it.

ANSWER: You're wrong. Sugar does not love you. Not according to all the studies that have come out recently about the deleterious effects sugar has on our health, such as diabetes, obesity, and heart disease just to name a few. I'm not asking you to cut out sugar completely from your diet—

QUESTION: Wait, hold on, me again, the sugar lover. Okay, okay, I get that you think sugar's "evil," but everything in moderation, right? I only eat, like, a piece of pie or cake on weekends with a little ice cream, maybe a handful of M&Ms in the afternoons or before I go to bed at night. That's not so bad, right?

ANSWER: That's a lot of sugar. And it may not be all the sugar you're eating. Do you read food labels? Americans still haven't recovered from the low-fat foods craze that started a few decades ago. Remember that? Low-fat cookies, rice cakes, milk, yogurt, ice cream, cheese, margarine, and on and on—all low in fat. What started that trend? Americans were suffering heart disease in record numbers, and the conclusion science and our government came to was that fat and cholesterol were the culprits. Naturally, therefore, if we cut our fat intake, we would reduce heart disease. Easy, right? And the food industry jumped in the fat-cutting waters, making a splash by sucking out the fat from our foods. But one production problem they encountered, predictably, is that most of food's flavor comes from fat. So how to make up for lost flavor? They pumped our yogurts and milks and cheeses and granola bars and breakfast cereals and snack foods full of sugar (along with some chemical additives for good measure). As a result of the low-fat craze, America's diabetes and obesity rates exploded, and not surprisingly, our hearts didn't get any healthier. That's why the FDA reversed itself a few years ago and told us, sure, okay, go ahead and add some whole fats back into your diet. But there's still a lot of sugar out there you may not even know you're eating. That's why it's important to read food labels.

QUESTION: **How many carbs should I eat a day?**

ANSWER: Eat carbs according to the intensity of your output.

- During base-building periods and on rest days eat around 100 to 150 grams of carbs.

- On high-intensity training days eat 150 to 200 grams of carbs.

QUESTION: **What about portion size?**

ANSWER: That's an important question, because even the healthiest foods like broccoli and kale, if cooked in oil, become high-fat, high-calorie. Which is actually the goal—to make them healthy but filling. But no matter how healthy they are, if you eat too much of them, you'll gain weight. So what calculus do I use to determine portion size? I don't use math. There's too many factors to determine such as age, gender, activity level, weight, metabolism. One size doesn't fit all. Besides, do you really want to weigh all your food or count every calorie you eat?

I prefer a more intuitive approach, one that builds food awareness. First, eat only when you're hungry. Second, eat as much as you need and no more. Pay attention to how you full you're getting, and stop before you get too full. You win no awards for being a Clean Plate Ranger. Save those extra Brussels sprouts and that grilled swordfish for tomorrow's lunch. Never walk away from a meal stuffed.

But you should know the nutritional percentages of your diet in terms of fats, protein, and carbohydrate intake. On days when you do low-intensity cardio or no exercise at all:

- 65 percent fats, 20 percent protein, and 15 percent carbohydrates like sweet potatoes, quinoa, and brown rice.

During high-intensity workout days the percentages shift to allow more carbs:

- 60 percent fats, 20 percent protein, and 20 percent carbs.

QUESTION: **Don Johnson said something about food input and cardio output speaking to each other. What does that mean?**

ANSWER: Wouldn't it be the coolest thing in the world if we could eat a certain kind of food, like fats, and then do a certain kind of exercise, such as low-intensity cardio that burned those fats almost exclusively for fuel so the body would be in perfect sync? If that could happen, it would be the most efficient energy burning system ever devised. Well, that's what happens when you become adapted to a healthy-fats diet and do low-intensity cardio exercise. That's what Don means when he says, "our food input and output talking to each other." I'll go into it in greater detail in the next chapter, Cardio, but you'll begin your cardio training by doing low-intensity cardio that uses fat for its fuel, so from now on your body will be learning to tap into your fat reserves to fuel it. And then later, when you add high-intensity cardio into the mix, you'll add more carbs, the fuel your body asks for when it's working hard in short bursts. The bigger picture is that I'm going to teach you how to eat based on your activity level, including those days when you don't have time to get any exercise.

QUESTION: I put Stevia in my coffee in the mornings and sometimes use it to sweeten baked foods. Your diet is plant based and Stevia's a plant, so that's okay, right?

ANSWER: Stevia might be better than eating sugar, but I don't like substitutes. They're crutches, Band-Aids, and you should wean yourself off of them. They're also subject to abuse. For instance, you bake with Stevia? What do you bake? Cookies, pies, cakes, scones, donuts? See where I'm going? The other thing about all sweeteners is that their ubiquity has dulled our palates. We've become so normalized to oversweetened foods that we sometimes don't appreciate the simplicity and wonder of purer, unadulterated foods.

I hope I've answered a lot of your questions. But let's face it: no two people have the same schedules or the same food likes and dislikes, so you will have to figure some things out on your own. But to get an idea of what a healthy-fats diet can look like on a daily basis, let's go through a typical day in my boring life, one meal at a time.

BREAKFAST

To me the old adage about breakfast being the most important meal of the day hits the mark, at least from a nutritional standpoint. It's a great way to get on track from the start, or at least get one meal right in case the rest of the day goes to hell. (Hey, it happens to the best of us.) Also, when you eat good fats in the morning your energy levels stay even all day, so you can focus and get your shit done. A few days a week, I make a two-egg omelet with avocado, onions, peppers, and spinach, whole-grain toast, and some berries. Be creative with your veggies: an omelet is an easy enough dish to master, so you can play around with spices and all kinds of veggies. Or, I eat leftovers from my previous night's dinner. Chicken breast or other lean meat, vegetables, sweet potato or quinoa. On high-intensity training days when I need more carbs I eat oatmeal with ground flax and chia seeds with a scoop of protein powder. If that sounds like a lot of calories, well, it is—that's the point: it's dense, nutrient-rich food that satisfies.

PORTION CONTROL

As you're experimenting with these new ingredients, have fun, but be mindful of portion sizes. Some of my clients start their healthy-fats diet by wolfing down six eggs, five strips of bacon, and two avocados. No. Too much of a good thing isn't a good thing. Eat until you're satiated and no more.

Now, maybe you don't have the time to scramble a few eggs and sauté some veggies in the morning (tip: I cook my veggies the night before and simply reheat them). I get it, but you can still eat a healthy breakfast. I leave the house at 4:30 a.m. three days a week to train clients in Los Angeles, and on those mornings I make a smoothie with almond milk, coconut oil, spinach, protein powder, and berries. It's the perfect combination of good fats, veggies, and protein (and the berries add a tad of fiber) that powers me through until lunch.

LUNCH

Although your energy level is still high from your breakfast, you may be feeling the first hunger pangs for lunch. Or not. If that's the case, skip it; maybe have some almonds later on. The point is: don't eat unless you're hungry. But if you are hungry, let's talk lunch. Lunch shouldn't be as big as breakfast. The idea is to taper your input as the day goes on. I don't have time to sit down for lunch most days, so I'm a huge fan of organic salad bars in markets. I build a base of spinach, arugula, and other lettuces; add garbanzo beans, quinoa or brown rice, tomatoes, a few ounces of lean meat like grilled chicken breast or tuna, maybe a few olives, cucumbers, broccoli, and cauliflower; and dress it with olive oil, vinegar, and salt and pepper. Remember, unless it's a high-intensity training day, go light on the carbs. Salad bars are a great opportunity to experiment with different kinds of nutrients, but it's easy to pile it on, so beware of portion size.

If I'm eating out for lunch, I'll typically order a salad with a grilled chicken breast or, if they have it, wild salmon, and I'll ask for olive oil and vinegar as a dressing. If I don't see a similar salad on the menu, I'll ask if another dish can be simplified to include just the protein, veggies, and healthy fats. If I'm really stuck and end up with carbs on my plate, so be it—I eat a limited amount, drink loads of water, and move on.

DINNER

When it comes to family, social interaction, and just plain winding down from a busy day, dinner is often the biggest meal of the day. But when it comes to portion size, it should be the smallest. Try to focus your dinners around high-quality food—your very favorites— but in very small portions. I usually serve two or three kinds of vegetables along with four to five ounces of salmon, or three ounces of grass-fed beef, bison, or chicken and a small amount of carbs. I find that if I eat too much for dinner, the next morning I'm not hungry for breakfast, that most important meal, and my whole eating cycle is thrown askew. Make dinner special and savor every bite. Just eat smaller portions.

Your busy schedule, lifestyle, and personal tastes are likely different from mine, and I encourage you to be creative and have fun when it comes to planning your meals. The best way to take control of how you eat is to shop for and cook your own meals. Maybe you have a busy schedule and that's not possible. Or you think it's not. I'll give you some tips about how Kelly and I pull it off with our busy schedules later when you start making changes to your diet. But to get you started thinking about it for the next time you go food shopping, here are two lists, one of foods you should start filling your diet with and the other of the ones you should begin avoiding.

DO FOODS

- **EGGS.** A miracle food loaded with good fats and protein. I eat them two to four times per week, and my HDL is 144 and my LDL is 86. Triglycerides? 78.

- **FISH.** Choose fatty fish like wild salmon, anchovy, sardines, oysters, mussels, or wild-caught shrimp.

- **MEAT.** Try to buy organic or grass fed, not processed. Organic means no hormones or antibiotics and the animals are fed organic grains and graze in pastures, not feed lots. Sure, in addition to being more humane and better for the environment, grass-fed beef and bison are high in omega-3s, so it's healthier for you too.

- **DAIRY.** Use sparingly. Buy organic butter, cream, goat cheese, and whole-fat yogurt. If you buy low- or no-fat dairy, it typically has added sugar, as fat is what gives dairy its flavor.

- **NONDAIRY MILKS.** Try to stick to unsweetened nut milks like cashew and almond. I actually prefer the taste of almond milk to cow's milk.

- **VEGETABLES.** Spinach, lettuce, kale, chard, cauliflower, onion, and broccoli. But again, it's hard to go wrong with veggies.

- **NUTS.** Choose macadamia and almonds, but sparingly.

- **FRUITS.** Tomatoes and avocados are technically fruits, though we don't treat them as such. But eat them—they're great for you. Also eat grapefruit, blueberries, raspberries, strawberries, blackberries, and apples. But absolutely stay away from fruit juices: they're all the sugar and none of the fiber.

- **TEA AND COFFEE.** Flavor with full-fat dairy if you like, but no added sugar.

- **HEALTHY FAT OILS.** Extra virgin olive oil is the most common and found in almost every grocery store. Avocado oil is great to use in cooking because it doesn't burn or lose its healthy properties at high temperatures when you're sautéing all those veggies. Coconut oil is also a great choice.

- **CARBOHYDRATES.** Sweet potatoes, quinoa, rice, fruits—but all in small portions. What's small? Twenty percent or less of your whole menu. One measurement that might help is, for women, keep your rice, quinoa, and sweet potatoes to as much as you can cup in your hand. For men, you get one to two handfuls.

DON'T FOODS

- **SUGAR.** As I stated earlier, I don't add sugar to anything and eat nothing to which sugar is added, except high-cocoa (80% or higher), low-sugar dark chocolate.

- **ARTIFICIAL SWEETENERS.** As I said before, they're crutches and you should wean off of them.

- **BREAD.** Bread is pure carbs, no way around that. But if you're going to eat bread, seek out naturally leavened, whole-grain bread. Or sprouted grain bread such as Ezekiel Bread. Also, bread fermented naturally (using wild, not commercial yeasts) has been proven to have beneficial health qualities for the gut and is consumed by many societies with populations that live the longest. But absolutely stay away from grocery store, sliced bread. Why? Bread should be flour, water, yeast, and salt. Store-bought bread has ingredient lists longer than a Tolstoy novel.

- **PASTA.** God, I love pasta. With a spicy tomato sauce or clams or lots of mixed vegetables and shrimp, but—just three-quarters of a cup of De Cecco Fusilli has a whopping forty-one grams of carbs. That just kills me. But you don't have to give up pasta entirely. Want pasta primavera (pasta with vegetables)? Go for it. But instead of having the traditional bowl full of pasta with a few vegetables on top, fill the bowl with vegetables (that have been cooked in olive oil and garlic), and add a little pasta on top—say, a quarter of a cup. You can also add fish or chicken into the mix—or better yet, crack an egg over it all and let it cook in. Then grate some fresh cheese on top, and that's a damn tasty, low-carb meal.

- **BREAKFAST CEREALS, AND PASTRIES (MUFFINS, CROISSANTS, BAGELS, DONUTS).** No. Just don't. Stay away. Like soda, these are all pure sugar and/or carb bombs.

- **CANDY.** 'Nuff said.

- **DESSERTS.** If you have a major sweet tooth and can't ignore dessert, buy some high-quality dark chocolate and break off a few small squares as your after-dinner treat. The higher the percentage of cocoa, the lower the amount of sugar. I munch on Valrhona's 85 percent chocolate bars, which have only three grams of sugar per serving. It takes some getting used to, but after purging most sugar from your diet, you'll appreciate the slightly bitter but satisfying treat.

NUTRITION SUMMARY

> Eating healthy fat foods is a return to eating the way your grandparents ate, back before diabetes, obesity, and other food diseases were even an issue.

> Eat carbs based on your exercise intensity output. On days when you do high-intensity training you should aim for 150 to 200 grams of carbs per day. On base-building and sedentary days eat 100 to 150 grams of carbs per day or less.

> Avoid sugar and processed foods.

> Eat real food, including vegetables, eggs, lean meats, nuts, healthy-fat and oils.

> To take the guess work out of your food intake, consider using one of the cool new apps like My Macros+ or MyFitnessPal. These apps keep track of your total calories consumed as well as macronutrients—fat, protein, and carbohydrates. At just a glance, you can see where you stand nutrition-wise today, this week, this month—and beyond.

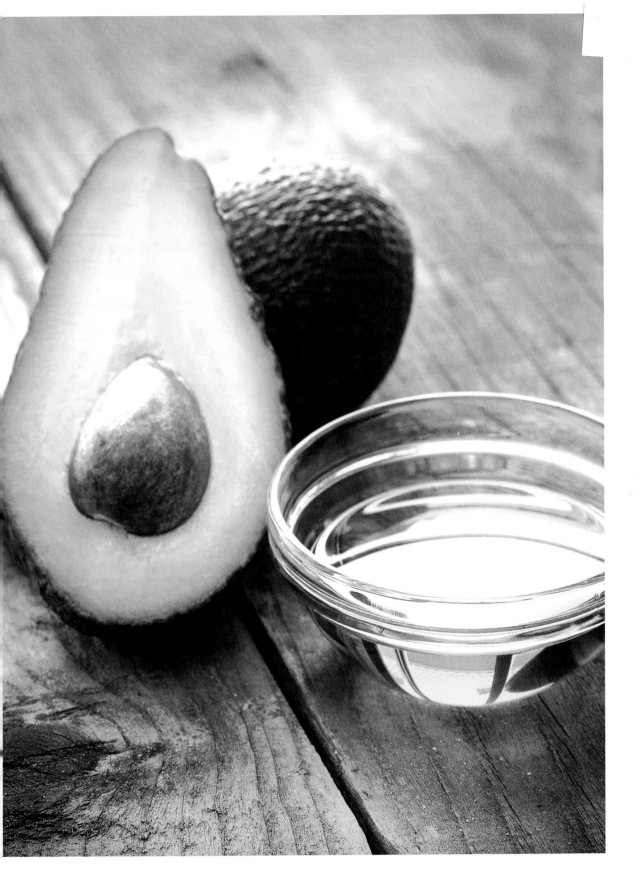

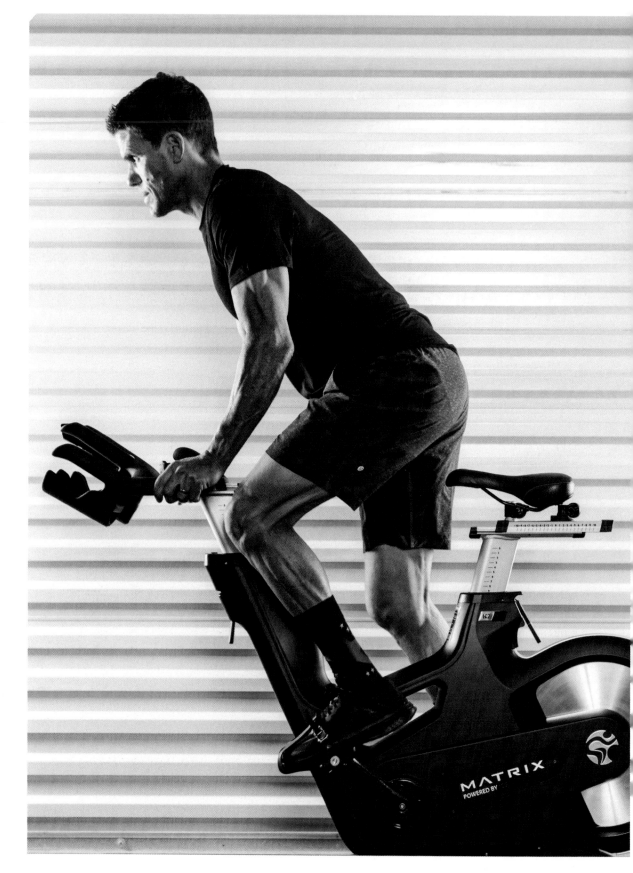

CHAPTER TWO: CARDIO

SWITCHING TO A HEALTHY-FAT, plant-centric diet—putting the right fuel in your tank—is the first step on your journey. The next step is teaching your body how to use its new primary fuel source. And you're going to do that by performing low-intensity cardiovascular exercise, which will, at the same time, start rebuilding your base level of aerobic fitness. Once you've built that foundation, you'll be well on your way toward rebounding.

I want to start by explaining why cardio is so important. Human beings are born to move. We have long limbs, a big brain, and a uniquely upright, bipedal body, all so we can scan the horizon and contemplate and execute our next important—*move.* Our ancestors made good use of their abilities. They spent their days hunting (walking, jogging, sprinting, crawling) and gathering (climbing, digging, squatting) their food, building shelters, and making tools and clothes. And while all those activities exercised most of their bodies' muscles, constant movement also raised their heart rate—the number of times the heart beats per minute (as we measure it today). Raising the heart rate causes the heart to pump more blood, oxygenating the body, expending energy, burning off stress and fat, and strengthening the heart.

In other words, while cardio exercise works a lot of the muscles in the body, the most important muscle it works is your heart. And your heart is the most important muscle in your body. Ergo, cardio exercise truly matters.

ON HATING CARDIO
By Mike Kelley

I've always hated cardio. Even way back in high school. I just wasn't good at it. I'm more fast twitch and explosive—not like Peter, the Energizer Bunny who could go for forever. When I first started training alongside Chip and John I did pretty well at the strength stuff, but when we got to the cardio at the end of the workout they trounced me. Both of them are endurance guys from way back, and it was clear I'd never be able to hang with them, so I decided to give up. But Peter said before I quit I should try coming into the gym on off days and do longer, low-intensity cardio to build up my aerobic base. He said going slow for some people is tough and that I'd have to check my ego at the gym door, but if I kept at it, I'd eventually see gains. As much as I hated doing cardio on machines, I went in to Platinum two to three days a week and did long, slower cardio on the SkiErg and bike. Over the first few weeks I started seeing some improvement. That sparked motivation, and I didn't mind the workouts so much anymore. Pretty soon I started catching up to Chip and John and then hanging with them. No one was more surprised than me. I guess that's part of getting older. Getting out of stuck places, seeing yourself differently, and finding out you don't suck at things you thought you did—hopefully before it's too late.

Our ancestors were great at doing natural cardio workouts as part of their daily lives—digging for roots, climbing for fruit, running after prey—and sometimes running from predators! But modern man is not. We sit most of the day, and that means our heart rate beats at its resting rate, never being challenged, neglected like a dog who wants nothing more than to be taken out for a walk or run. But I get it. You don't have time, right? Work, family, social obligations—there's always some excuse. And the one I hear most: "I hate doing cardio on machines." If you detest running on a treadmill, cycling on a stationary bike, doing the elliptical—or even getting up off the damn sofa—I'm speaking directly to you now. I get it. I really do. But just think about what might happen to you if you keep neglecting your heart over time. Maybe you don't want to face that truth. Keep reading and I'll tell you about someone else who didn't want to face it either, one of my longtime clients, "Ben."

LOW-INTENSITY CARDIO TRAINING

"You gotta go slow to get fast!"

Ben was a successful businessman who spent twenty-five years working day and night at his desk. Over time eighty pounds crept on his frame, his blood work scared his doctor, and everything hurt when he moved. So he simply stopped moving. A former college football player, Ben remembered what it *felt like* to move well and do whatever he wanted, and his sedentary state depressed him. He took prescription drugs for pain, but his unhappiness was taking a toll on him and his family. So he decided to make a change. He quit his job and moved his family to Santa Barbara to start over.

A doctor who'd been helping Ben with his back problems connected me with him. The first thing I advised Ben to do was switch his animal-fat-loaded, processed, high-carb diet to a healthy-fats diet, which he did immediately. Ben's that kind of guy who can turn the switch and, boom, he's all in. The next step was teaching Ben's body how to burn those fats and build a base level of fitness—cardiovascular exercise. But that was more of a challenge. Ben was in awful shape. His resting heart rate was in the high 80s, his blood pressure was beyond high—as they say, he was a heart attack waiting to happen. And he had old injuries that plagued him because he'd lost so much muscle strength. He couldn't even walk on the treadmill without pain. I didn't want to put him on the bike either: he sat all day long and would just be reinforcing his bad posture.

So I started Ben on the elliptical. He's a sharp, inquisitive man, the kind of guy who asks questions every step of the way. "How fast should I go?" he asked.

Low-intensity, aerobic cardio equals about 65 to 75 percent of your maximum exertion, and that's where I wanted him to stay for the first four or so weeks.

"I have no clue how to determine 65 to 75 percent," Ben said. He's not alone: most people don't. The best way to measure your exertion or output level is by monitoring your heart rate. Ben needed to move as fast or as slow as was necessary to get to and hold his MAHR.

"What the hell's a MAHR?" Ben asked. Another good question! MAHR is your *maximum aerobic heart rate*, the target number of beats per minute your heart should pound during low-intensity, aerobic cardio exercise.

"Why's that so important?" Ben queried. When you do low-intensity exercise you burn fat as fuel—the same fats you're now fueling your body with. Or as Don Johnson put it, you're getting your input (food) and your output (cardio) to talk to each other. Doing low-intensity cardio also builds base fitness, which Ben didn't have yet.

"So how do I know what my MAHR is?" Ben followed up with. That's easy. Using Phil Maffetone's MAHR formula, take your age and subtract it from 180. Ben was 50 then, so his MAHR was 130. How did Ben know when his heart was hitting 130 beats per minute? I slapped a heart rate monitor on him. If you don't have a heart rate monitor, I suggest you invest in one. (You may already own one if you have a step counter like the Fitbit or the Apple watch.) Numbers don't lie, and using a heart rate monitor will let you precisely track your progress and take the guesswork out of your cardio workouts.

PERCEIVED EXERTION

If you don't want to buy or use a heart rate monitor, you can approximate your MAHR by feel or *perceived exertion*. Perceived exertion is only a guesstimate, but if you're mindful of how hard you're working—or not working—you'll at least come close to achieving your MAHR. Here are a few indicators you've reached your MAHR, or 65 to 75 percent of your max output, during cardio: you're breathing pretty hard, sweating, and yet you're still able to hold a conversation.

As you start to get fitter, you'll begin moving faster while holding your MAHR. For instance, when Ben started on the elliptical he generated 100 to 110 watts of power to reach his 130 MAHR and could only hold it for about ten minutes. But within three weeks he was generating 125 to 140 watts at his 130 MAHR and holding it for twenty to twenty-five minutes. By the end of his first four weeks his body had learned how to use fat as fuel, and he had built a solid fitness base, holding 170 to 200 watts for thirty to forty minutes.

For the first four weeks you'll do only low-intensity cardio like Ben did and slowly build back your aerobic base. Some people get bored with base building and mistakenly believe that if they go faster (pedal the bike harder, row the rower quicker, pump the elliptical faster), they'll get back in shape quicker. Not true. In fact, going hard at the beginning is how people get injured. Also, going just a bit harder (but still short of high intensity) means entering the "no man's land" that exists between low-intensity and high-intensity cardio training in which you're working pretty hard but your heart makes very few gains. It's just inefficient. *You gotta go slow to get fast.* So grab your headphones and find a cool podcast or cue up your favorite tunes, and learn to appreciate low-intensity, base-building cardio exercise. Don't worry: soon enough you'll graduate to the harder stuff just like Ben did.

INTERVAL TRAINING

After four weeks of base building I started mixing in some intervals into Ben's workout and, of course, increased his carb intake on his training days. You may have heard of interval training before. Ben had done intervals as a college athlete. Intervals are not new or exotic, but once you've built a solid cardio base, they will take you to higher levels of cardio fitness faster than any other kind of cardio. And intervals will also help you lose weight because of the "afterburn" effect: you've worked so hard that your metabolism is elevated long after your workout is over.

What exactly are intervals? The folks at Merriam-Webster define the word *interval* pretty succinctly: "A period of time between events." For our purposes *events* are both a period of ON time when you exercise at a high rate of exertion and a period of OFF time when you recover just enough so you can go ON again. We talked about how the heart is a muscle, just like your quadriceps, bicep, or pectorals. What's the best way to make your quads, biceps, or pecs fitter? By doing multiple reps and sets of exercises with a period of ON time between events and a period of OFF time too. The heart muscle works the same way. You work your heart hard by doing a short burst of exercise on the bike, treadmill or rower, then let your heart recover between events. That's one set.

The following is a sample interval training session. Note that where the expression "x" follows a number, "x" means times, as in the number of times you will do the interval or the number of times you rest afterward.

> ## WARM-UP

- 1 minute of easy effort (60–75 percent effort)

- 1 minute easy, 2x 30 seconds 80 percent effort, with 30 seconds off in between sets.

> ## MAIN SET

- 1x 2 minutes at 80 to 85 percent effort, 2 minutes off in between. (In other words, do 2 minutes on, then take 2 minutes off.)

- 2x 1 minute at 85 percent effort, 1 minute off. (In other words, do 1 minute at 85 percent, rest for 1 minute, another 1 minute on, then another 1 minute rest.)

- 3x 30 seconds at 90 to 95 percent effort, 30 seconds off in between. (In other words, do 30 seconds on, and take 30 seconds off, 3 times.)

> COOL-DOWN

- Cool down is a 2-minute, post-interval period of pedaling, skiing, climbing, or walking at a very slow pace to bring your heart rate back down over time.

If you did the math, you noticed that the interval session above takes only about fifteen to twenty minutes to complete. And that's what Ben appreciated most about intervals: like circuit training, the workouts are super-efficient—"The most bang for the buck," as he put it. Ben appreciates a challenge. He'd built a good cardio base, so he was pretty damn happy to start interval training. And pretty soon really great things started happening for Ben. He'd lost weight, was moving well again without pain, and was building good muscle strength. Interval training was what truly jump-started his rebound back to being fit.

QUESTION: Should I train on the cardio machines in my gym, or should I go outside and run or cycle?

ANSWER: On the weekends or when you have time, I encourage you to go outside for a run, a hike, a bike ride—whatever, just get a good long, easy one in. But for your gym sessions the best, most efficient way to get your workouts done is to do your cardio right there in the gym. Cardio comes right after strength circuits, there's no down time in between, so you need to get at it. Also, cardio machines help you track your progress: they can measure your output (watts, rpms, strides per minute, etc.) and time, speed and distance (how long, how fast, how far.) Along with a heart rate monitor, you can use all that data to make sure you're hitting all your targets and measure your progress.

QUESTION: Cardio machines are so boring. Any tricks you've learned to make them interesting enough so I don't want to blow my brains out?

ANSWER: Listening to podcasts during low-intensity cardio and music during high-intensity training keep me from killing myself on cardio machines! Nothing powers me through intervals better than Metallica. Another trick is to cross-train—go from one machine to another. That keeps things lively. All that said, however, and I don't mean to be a hard-ass here, but cardio training is as much a mental exercise as a physical one. If you're keeping track of your heart rate, watts, or RPMs, if you're diligent about making sure your posture is strong, and if you're challenging yourself to go a little bit harder every time you train, like Mike Kelley did—that challenge should hold your interest.

QUESTION: Which cardio machines are the best?

ANSWER: There is no "best"—there's only what works best for you. For instance, Ben sat on his ass at work all day, so I wasn't about to let him sit on the bike, right? If you have any lower back pain, stay away from the rower. If you experience knee pain, the Concept 2 SkiErg, the Airdyne, stationary bike, or an elliptical machine should work for you. If your gym has a Versa Climber, that's my favorite machine. I like to alternate back and forth between the Versa and the Concept 2 SkiErg. That's a killer workout, and both are great for doing intervals.

CARDIO MACHINES

One of the best machines overall is the elliptical. Not only do you get a good cardio workout that's very low impact, but if you hold onto the bars, you can actually create tension (which you'll learn about during Chapter Six: Tensioning for Strength) by packing down your shoulders and lats and working to build good posture. Be sure to keep your chin back and core activated and to push through the midfoot or heels, never the ball of your foot, or you'll put too much weight on the knees.

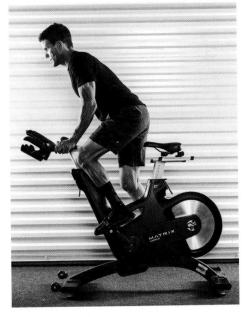

I also love indoor cycling. Sure, I'd rather be mountain biking in the backcountry, but that's not always possible. Be aware of your form: keep your knees from bowing outward, and keep your body still (don't flop all over the place), or you'll suffer what I call "power leaks" (your body's so loose and sloppy that the power's leaking out everywhere except where it should go: the pedals). Above all, focus on your posture. Your back should be flat as a board, with your shoulders packed down, not hunched up toward your ears. You can use the handlebars to create tension through your abs and upper torso so you're working your whole body.

If you have knee issues but are stubborn and want to run on the treadmill, raise the incline level so you're running "uphill." That moves the pounding force from the knees to the back of the legs. And use the opportunity to focus on your posture. Running with bad posture reinforces faulty patterns with every step you take, so be aware of your running posture (although don't let it prohibit you from running with a relaxed gait). Keep your eyes forward, chin up, and shoulders packed down.

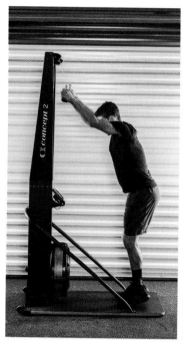
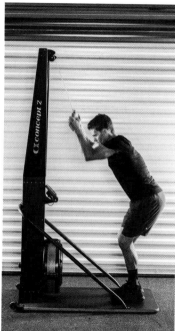
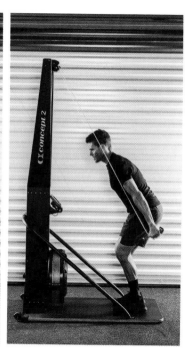

After I suffered a knee injury a few years ago I couldn't bike, run, or even do the elliptical, so I skied. And skied and skied and skied. A couple of times I did marathons. The Concept 2 SkiErg saved me during that dark time in my life. The SkiErg also helped reinforce my hinge pattern and worked my back, lats, glutes, and, more importantly, my heart. And I love doing intervals on the skier. If you have a partner, just pass the handles over to her or him at the end of your turn, recover, and go again. I can't say enough good things about this machine.

I have to admit I have a love-hate relationship with the Versa Climber because it's so challenging. Yet it will jack your heart rate up more quickly than any other machine. When you're on the Versa Climber, focus on bracing your core, and be sure to keep your shoulders packed down and maintain good posture.

CARDIO SUMMARY

> Cardio exercises the heart, helps burn fat and stress, and keeps the body fit.

> Do one longer cardio session on the weekend. Take it easy and make your bike ride, hike, or cross-country skiing enjoyable, not a chore.

> Low-intensity, base-building cardio exercise taps into your fat stores for energy. It's the perfect partner for the healthy-fats diet.

> High-intensity, interval training is what gives you top-end fitness, but it also taps into your glycogen or sugar stores for energy, and during the weeks you're doing intervals you'll add more grams of carbs to your diet.

> Any cardio machine in your gym will get your heart rate up to where you need it to go. Choose the machine based on your own preferences, including what feels right, and what keeps you motivated.

> A heart rate monitor is like having your own coach: it tells you the numbers, and you stick to them. It's the only way of making sure you're working out at the intensity you need to be.

> Stick to the percentages in the interval workouts. You will notice most are the "sweet spot" for the 75–85 percent range, with a few weeks here and there at 90–95 percent. Too much intensity can kill your progression. Obey the rules!

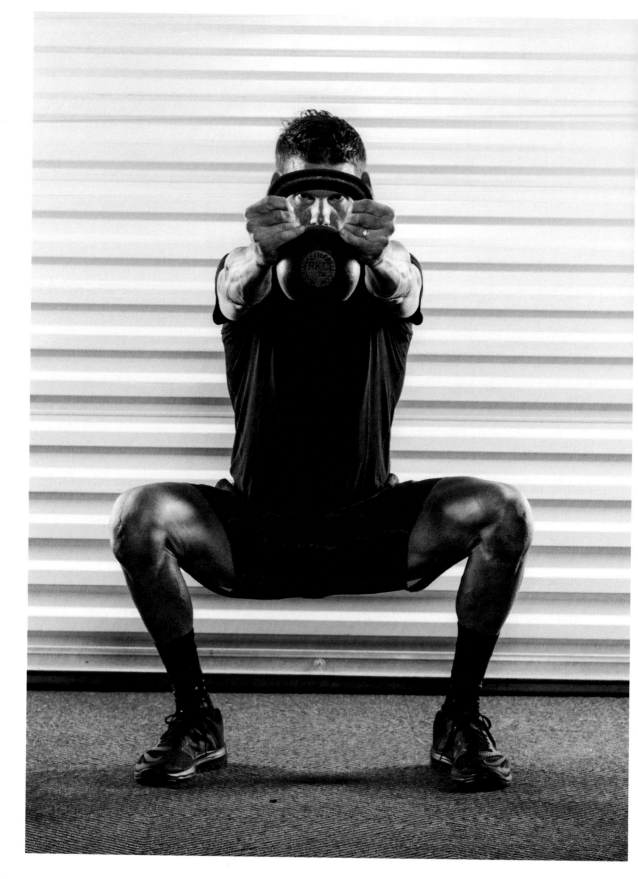

CHAPTER THREE: MOVEMENT

KEN ROCZEN IS ONE OF THE BEST athletes I've ever worked with. At just twenty-two, he has become one of the top Motocross and Supercross riders in the world. If you're not familiar with the sport of motocross racing, you might not understand why these riders have to train so hard. After all, it's not their body's engine that's propelling them but the bike's. But imagine spending thirty minutes with your heart rate maxed out while maintaining focus so you don't crash, all the while trying to control a high-powered, 250-pound motorcycle during a balls-out competition. You gotta be in damn good shape to pull it off.

Ken was so good at his sport that a lot of people expected he'd win both the Motocross and Supercross titles in 2016. But in May of 2015 he fractured his vertebrae. Ken kept racing, but he needed epidurals before races just to make it through. Incredibly, he ended the season in second place, but he was miserable and in pain. He considered having surgery, the only way to repair the fracture, but that meant sitting out his entire 2016 season. And Ken had a lot on the line. For one, his sponsors expected him to race—and to win. But on a more personal level Ken was a fierce competitor in his prime and didn't want to sacrifice an entire season. In a last-ditch effort his agent called me up, and I went down San Diego to see how I could help.

First thing I did with Ken was put him through some simple movements, and it quickly became clear why (besides his injury) he was in such a world of hurt. His body

UNDER WATER
By Chip Blankenhorn

By the time I was in my early twenties I'd spent a lifetime in the pool because, like most swimmers and water polo players, I dedicated most of my training to swimming laps. Sure, I did some weight lifting at Stanford with the water polo team, but I focused mostly on my upper-body strength, because that's what I needed for my sport. By the time I was done with school and was well into my career I was having trouble keeping fit on dry land. I tried running, but I got shin splints and pulled calf muscles. And as I got older my posture started sagging, my lower back hurt, and I'd gained some pounds. I kept saying I'll eventually do something about it, but I didn't. Why? Looking back, I didn't really know how. So when John Murphy called, I jumped at the chance to work with Peter. We started by doing movement practice, easy hinges, squats, and long holds, but I couldn't do them, not as well as John and Mike (who weren't so hot at it either). Frustrated, I asked Peter, "What gives?"

"Chip," he said, "swimming's a great way to build cardio and muscle endurance, but if that's all you do, it's like you're living in a zero-gravity environment, and we don't live in outer space. Your body just doesn't know how to move right on dry land."

Encouraging, right? But a month of movement practice later, and everything changed. I was moving pretty good—well enough that Peter began having me lift weights. That's when I got really strong. John can kick my ass on the bike and Versa Climber, but strength stuff, like the SkiErg and pushing the sled, that's my domain. But it all started with learning how to move again.

had adapted to his back injury by developing new movement patterns around the injury. But adapting doesn't mean getting out of pain; it just means the body has found a new way to keep on moving at any cost.

Of course, I couldn't fix Ken's fractured vertebrae, but I told him that if we could get him moving correctly again and then strengthen the posterior chain that supports the lower back, maybe it would diminish his pain. With his doctor's approval, we would try to get him back to a level of fitness that would hopefully mean he could race in the 2016 season. Ken was game and asked, "So where do we start?" The same place I start all my clients, I told him, and exactly where you'll start: Movement Practice to retrain faulty patterns.

A key concept behind Foundation Training is that it reteaches the body what it has forgotten over the years, which is how to move right again. Proper movement sets the stage for real fitness. Without it you're probably going nowhere, except maybe to your doctor. Once you've learned the movements in Chapter Seven and have achieved a proficient level, you'll begin adding weight and getting strong.

For example, during Movement Practice you'll learn a *hip hinge*. Once you're hinging well, you'll add weight, and that hinge becomes a *dead lift*, and a dead lift builds terrific glute and hamstring strength—and helps you learn the hinging pattern of the *kettlebell swing*, another good posterior chain exercise. A Foundation Training mainstay, the *woodpecker*, with added weight, becomes a *single-leg dead lift*. A *body weight squat* becomes a *goblet* and then a *Bulgarian split squat*. Progression, progression, progression. But it all starts with learning to move right again.

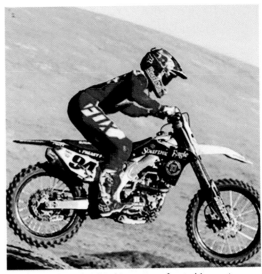

Ken Roczen's perfect hip hinges transfers to his sport.

And so I began Movement Practice with Ken. We focused on doing seven movements and Ken did them every day along with some low-intensity, base-rebuilding cardio. After three weeks Ken was moving well enough to progress to adding weight—or loading the patterns. For instance, he had been doing a body weight squat for three weeks to remaster the pattern and to regain lost mobility. When he could squat well again, keeping his heels flat on the ground, his back flat, not rounded, and rising up with some explosiveness, I front-loaded Ken with a kettlebell (as you will too) to perform the same movement, which is called a *goblet squat*. And the *wide founder* that was key to correcting his posture and reactivating his sleepy glutes became a *wide founder row*, which works the lats and upper back specifically, but engages the whole body to perform the movement.

Like Ken, you'll learn the movements, practice them until you have retrained your body to perform them correctly, and then—and only then—you'll add weight to the movements to build strength. Movement, progress, add weight, progress, get stronger, progress—that's how the program works.

And things were progressing well for Ken, so he decided to move to Santa Barbara for the winter to train with me. After about a month we started mountain biking up Romero Canyon to rebuild his cardio endurance. After two months Ken got back on the motorcycle and started riding again. He still had some pain here and there, but it was no longer debilitating. We continued to train as he prepared for the 2016 season.

The real test came in the winter of 2016, at the start of the indoor Supercross season.

Ken did pretty well in his first few races, but once he realized his back wasn't restricting him anymore, his confidence came flooding back and he dominated the final races at the end of the season and placed second overall. Next up was outdoor Motocross, in which the races are twice as long and twice as demanding. Ken completely dominated that season, winning twenty out of twenty-four races and claiming the championship by a landslide. He is now the best motocross rider in the world.

(Ken Roczen update, during the writing of this book: After winning the first two races of the 2017 Supercross season Ken crashed in the third, shattering all the bones in his left arm, wrist, and hand. He's had eight operations to reconstruct the bones, carti-lage, ligaments, tendons—the whole arm. He knows his comeback is going to be a long, uphill march. And the first step he'll take when he returns to training will be movement practice all over again.)

Ken's an extreme example of what happens when your body learns to move right again. But my three successful guinea pigs, John, Chip, and Mike, all did the exact same program, and they're all back to being active and playing the sports they love. The same is true for the pro athletes I train and the young moms looking to get back in shape. I even trained an oil tycoon whose back pain prevented him from doing the activity he loved most—playing golf—because his movement patterns were shot. Teaching him how to move correctly again and rebuilding his strength got him back on the links.

Whatever your fitness goals are, this book will help you learn how to move again, create a solid foundation on which to build real strength, regain good posture, and prog-ress your way forward.

QUESTION: I've had back pain for several years and would like to try your movement program, but I'm afraid doing movement practice might hurt my back. I don't want to make it worse. What should I do?

ANSWER: What does your doctor say? You should always get your doctor's okay before you start any new exercise program. But to answer your question, have you suffered a serious back injury such as a ruptured or torn disc or a pinched nerve or herniated disc that might require surgery? A serious injury requires serious treatment. However, if you have chronic, low-level, pain-in-the-ass, lower back pain from sitting too much, poor posture, faulty movement patterns, or overuse at work, Foundation exercises can help you overcome your pain.

QUESTION: I danced ballet for twenty years, and though it's been awhile and I am out of shape, my posture's still stick-straight and I think I still move really well. Won't Foundation and movement practice be a waste of time for me?

ANSWER: I've trained some of the best professional athletes in the world, many of them blow me away with what they can do. And yet I'd say 95 percent of them when they first start working with me have faulty movement patterns. It's just human nature—or maybe a modern-day affliction. You have to work at it—and keep working at it as you get older, because things will only get worse if you don't. I still do movement practice almost every day, so no, I don't think it's a waste of time at all.

MOVEMENT SUMMARY

> Everything starts with proper movement, which then becomes the start of building fitness and strength.

> The *Rebound* workout is all about progression: learn the movement, add weight to the pattern, then learn more movements. That's how you get strong, step by step.

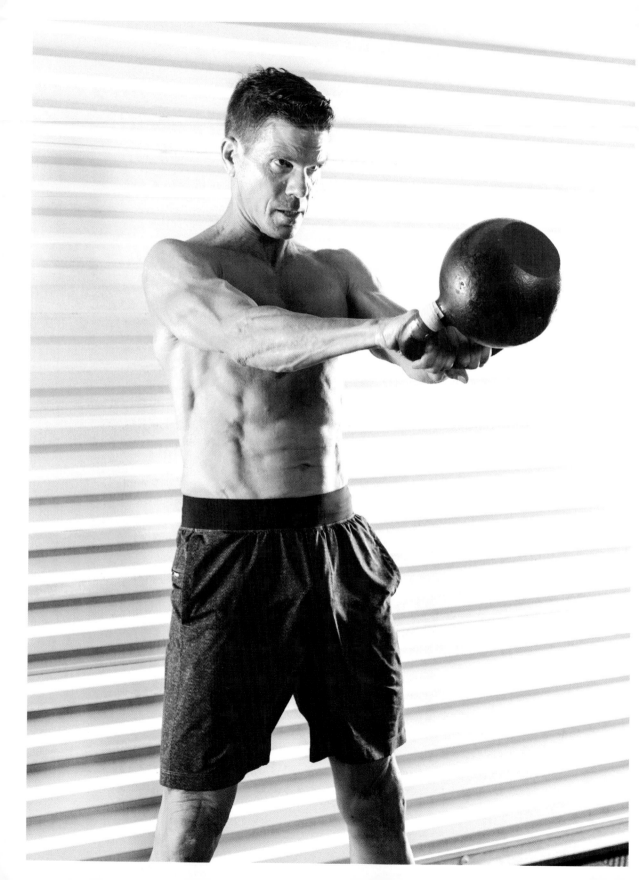

CHAPTER FOUR: STRENGTH

> ## The Fountain of Youth

ALL THREE PARTS OF THE REBOUND WORKOUT I've talked about so far—Nutrition, Cardio, and Movement—are valuable and potentially transformative on their own. If you followed my nutrition advice and returned to eating real, simple foods again and did nothing else in this book, the price of admission would have been worth it—cutting out sugar and processed foods will no doubt help improve your health, make you shed a few pounds, and increase your energy and confidence. If you only did the thirty or so cardio workouts printed in the pages that follow, you'd get in pretty damn good cardiovascular shape—the key to heart health, stress relief, and overall fitness. And movement? If all you do is movement practice, you'll get your body moving right again, improve your posture, and alleviate nagging pain.

And yet the most important part of your Rebounding is getting strong again. Why? Strength training truly is the fountain of youth.

BARRY BEING BARRY

In 1991, when I was still racing Ironman competitions, I met Barry Cappello, a high-power trial attorney then in his early fifties. At work, play, sport—in every part of his life—Barry gives every ounce of himself. When it comes to exercise, back then Barry had been racing marathons. He loves to compete. But all his years of sitting behind a desk and all the miles he logged during training had teamed up to make him tight and inflexible,

PEDALING HOPE
By John Murphy

First, let me just say that the two surgeries I had on my knees and the two operations I had on my shoulders were 100 percent my fault. Foolishness. Or, I'd like to think, youthful exuberance. Except I wasn't that young when I got hurt. Way back when, I did some triathlons, even a couple of Ironmans just to challenge myself. Then came life: work, travel, work, extra pounds, kids, work, stress, middle age, and lots of lower back pain. And bad impulses. Like jumping up off the couch and running a marathon without training for it. That's how I got injured. Why it took me so long to realize the harm I was causing myself, I don't know. Maybe I just wanted to have it all. I needed help, so I called Peter. When Chip, Mike, and I started training together, Chip had trouble with the movement practice stuff, and Mike would practically kill himself trying to keep up with us doing cardio. Me? After all my injuries, I was so weak that I could barely do one pushup. And not a single pull-up. After spending four weeks doing movement practice we added weight to the exercises, and Chip and Mike got so strong so fast. Not me. It took me longer, thanks to my injuries, but after time my body got strong enough that the pain in my knees and shoulders all but disappeared. And now I'm running, cycling, skiing again like when I was younger. What Peter sells most to guys like me, Mike, and Chip? The hope that that part of our lives isn't over yet.

and that created imbalances. And those weaknesses expressed themselves through pain and injuries like his chronic Achilles tendonitis.

But Barry refused to give up competing, so he quit racing marathons and took up triathlons—cross-training, in other words. A smart decision, cutting down on the repetitive motion of running. And Barry being Barry, he wanted to master the sport, so he hired a professional triathlete to teach him: me. And when I say teach, I don't mean just write him workouts and send him on his way: Barry wanted to do the same workouts I was doing, and when time permitted, he wanted to do them with me. Barry was the first client to follow me in my own training. What I did in the water, on the bike, and on the trail, Barry did it too.

To a lot of people that might sound crazy. I was in my midtwenties, and my full-time job was training for my sport. Barry was twice my age and worked ten to twelve hours a day behind a desk. But Barry being Barry, he threw himself into his triathlon training full force, following me up and down steep hills like Sea Ranch, pedaling up Gibraltar, and swimming through choppy waters at East Beach.

And although Barry got cardio fit, he hit a wall in his training. His injuries kept nagging him, he couldn't recover quickly enough to train hard the next day, and honestly, I thought he just didn't look as healthy as he should for someone in such good shape. What was going on? You didn't need to be a genius to figure it out: Barry was fighting Father Time—and losing. After the age of thirty we start to lose lean body mass, our metabolism slows down, a lot of us start gaining weight, we get weaker, our posture starts failing, and testosterone levels fall. How do you combat all that? Can you combat all that—or any of it?

I knew one aspect of Barry's overall training program was lacking: strength training. He has worked mainly on his own doing loads of bench presses, bicep curls, leg presses, and extensions—slow, isolating exercises—and while he looked strong, he wasn't, not functionally anyway. He was lifting the same way bodybuilders lift—the same way most people in gyms around the world still lift. I knew from my own experience that lifting that way didn't increase performance. And Barry wanted to perform. So I convinced him to let me be his trainer inside the gym too.

We started with the most basic exercises: squats, dead lifts, pushups, and lunges, and we focused on technique. What most people don't recognize is that weight lifting is a highly technical discipline that takes practice to perfect. Barry didn't have good technique at all—he'd never been taught to. In just a few months his imbalances disappeared, and so did his injuries. He got so strong so fast that we started lifting together. To this day Barry is still my workout partner.

Barry's seventy-four now, and he's still my equal in nearly every lift we do. He still runs, cycles, and swims, and every year on his birthday he and I go off for several days on a mountain biking trip, and he still kills it. And he hasn't suffered a significant injury and is stronger today than he was thirty years ago. He dead lifts twice his body weight and could easily join me, Chip, John, and Mike for a punishing Saturday morning work-out. His hormone levels are that of a thirty-five-year-old, his cholesterol and triglycerides are a doctor's dream, and he looks amazing. And that's because he got strong. Building strength enabled him to build all-around fitness. It made him able. And when you're able, you can do anything you want to. And Barry does.

Barry's just one example—and one of my favorites. But I've had so many clients experience similar transformations, proving that strength training truly is the fountain of youth. You can overcome pain, injury, and declining posture, and you can decrease the effects of osteoarthritis and other aging diseases if you get your body strong—and keep it that way.

QUESTION: Barry's story is inspiring, but I've heard some bad things about weight lifting over the years.

ANSWER: Many of my clients are dubious about weight lifting when they first start. And I understand why. Weight lifting has a rocky reputation, and somewhat deservedly so. Steroids, no pain no gain, giant muscles, injuries, crackpot trainers, six-minute workouts, bad practices, impossible dreams. Weight lifting is a science and a sport to be taken seriously, and I'm going to teach you how to do it right. If I accomplish nothing more in this book than to help you develop a love of lifting weights, then I will have succeeded.

QUESTION: But I'm a woman, and I don't want to get big muscles from lifting weights, so—?

ANSWER: I don't have big muscles, and neither does Barry or any of the trainers at Platinum. That's not what my program is for. What is it for? Let me tell you about one of my favorite people in the world, Diana Taurasi. Diana might be the best women's basketball player of all time. She's won three NCAA championships at UConn, four Olympic gold medals, rookie-of-the-year honor, and WNBA champion, and she holds a ton of scoring records. The NBA guys like Russell Westbrook and Al Horford have nothing but respect for her. As a guard she can shoot the lights out. And when you're that good at something, you want to do it for as long as you can. But as Diana got into her thirties, she couldn't recover after games and practices as quickly as she used to. She'd lost lean body mass, was injury prone, and knew she had lost a step. It was getting harder to keep up with the young kids coming into the league. She was feeling her age.

She didn't like strength training and, in fact, gave little merit to it, but every time I saw her at the basketball gym I'd get on her about it. Finally she agreed to let me take her through some training. She's such a good athlete and worked so hard, and after a month she was already getting stronger, and a lightbulb went off. She saw what she needed to do to stay competitive. And man, is she competitive. In 2016 she played in the Russia pro league and won the championship, got another Olympic gold in Rio, and played in the WNBA and hoped to win another championship there. (She didn't, but she was the league's leading scorer.) At age thirty-four, Diana's at the top of her game. And she hasn't put on one pound of bulk. She's long and lean. And thanks to giving up sugar and eating more healthy fats, she's lost some pounds. Diana's just one example. I've trained a lot of women and all have gotten stronger, and none have ever complained of getting bulky.

QUESTION: What exactly is circuit training?

ANSWER: Back when I was a bodybuilder I'd do a set of bench press, then stand around and shoot the shit with the guys for, like, five minutes while recovering before my next set. That recovery time is important. If the muscle you fatigued can't perform well during the next set, you won't build strength. But by the time I was done with five or six sets of bench press, a half an hour had passed, and the only thing I had to show for it was worked pecs. Not very efficient, to say the least. When I started training for Ironmans I needed to find a more efficient way to get strong.

Circuit training is all about time management. Instead of standing around waiting to recover, how can we use our time better? By working another muscle while the first one is recovering. And then work another and then maybe one more before coming back around to the first exercise and work that muscle again. For instance, in the Rincon workout you'll start Circuit One with Hinge Rows (lats, back), then do goblet squats (quads, glutes), then farmer carries (core, grip). You'll do that circuit three times through, then move on to the second circuit of dumbbell bench press (chest), single leg RDLs (hamstrings and glutes), and Turkish getups (everything!) By the time you've finished your circuits, you'll have worked most of the muscles in your body and in a very short amount of time.

You'll do the same circuits (with slight variations) for three weeks, and then I'll change the circuits around. Why three weeks? Three reasons: First, that's how long it takes to learn how to do the new movements correctly. Second, the human body adapts quickly to new stimuli, and after three weeks of shocking your muscles with new exercises, the shock wears off, the body adapts, and strength gains taper. So it's time to shock your body with new movement patterns. And lastly, most of my clients (me included) get bored of doing the same exercises after about three weeks, so to keep things interesting, you need to shake things up.

I've worked out a simple method of writing workouts for me and my clients over the years. Here's my language decoded:

- "Circuit One 2x" means do that entire circuit (of three to four exercises) all the way through, twice.

- Within an exercise, if I say "at 10x," that means do ten reps.

In week one you'll always learn new exercises, so you have to take it slower and lighter. You'll typically do circuits 2x (meaning the entire circuit all the way through, twice), using lighter weight at 10x (ten reps). In week two you'll do the circuits 3x using a heavier weight at 10x. In week three you'll do the circuits 3x using an even heavier weight at 8x. That's a general rule, although there will be some exceptions.

QUESTION: I've seen people using kettlebells at my gym. Those people do all kinds of elaborate movements with them. That intimidates me. And I know this sounds lame, but I don't want to look like an idiot in front of people. Can't I just stick with dumbbells?

ANSWER: You won't look like an idiot. A novice, perhaps, but I urge you to embrace the new adventure that is kettlebells. Why? Because when it comes to functional training, nothing is better. What is functional training? You're rebounding back to doing the everyday activities you want to do, like playing on the company softball team, cycling on weekends, planting your vegetable garden. Functional training mimics the movements you do to perform those activities, and exercises using kettlebells are the most functional kind of training there is. Why? The instability created during kettlebell exercises links muscles and muscle groups together and activates stabilizers to gain control of the weight. The more your body learns how to handle instability, the more stable and strong it becomes. In other words—and at the risk of sounding like a little, green Jedi—instability leads to stability, and stability leads to strength, and strength leads to your Rebound. And I'm going to teach you how to use kettlebells properly, so don't worry about what anyone thinks.

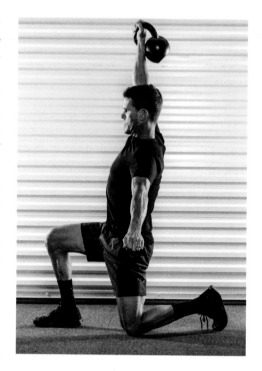

By the way, don't throw out your old friend the dumbbells yet. You're going to use them in this book too.

QUESTION: I tried doing kettlebell exercises, but the pressure on my wrist hurt too much. Solution?

ANSWER: Wear a sweat band (like tennis players wear) on your wrist, and it will take the pressure off.

QUESTION: Where do you stand with the old weight lifting adage, "No pain, no gain"?

ANSWER: I stand against it. Here's a new adage that I stole from Pavel, and I'm paraphrasing here: lifting to failure is failure. Why? Because form and technique are the most important aspects of lifting weights, and if you go to failure, you probably lost form two reps ago. Sure, work hard, but rather than kill yourself like I used to do back when I was young and foolish, I want you to master the form of each exercise, understand what it does for you, and fall in love with the art and science of weight training. Do that, and you'll stick to it the rest of your life.

QUESTION: How much weight should I use?

ANSWER: A good rule to follow is if you do the ascribed number of reps and could easily do one to two more, try going up in weight and see how it feels. But don't compromise your technique.

QUESTION: I'm sixty-five years old, and I've never lifted weights or played sports—I just want the pain in my knees and back to go away. But you're talking about kettlebells and instability and something called a Turkish whatever. Be honest: Is this workout really something I can even do?

ANSWER: Yes. But if you want to say, "Hey, Peter, screw your Turkish whatevers. They're just too damn complicated for me," I say good for you. I don't want you to do any exercise that makes you uncomfortable. But I don't want you to give up either. Instead, adapt. For instance, most anyone can do the first part of the Turkish getup known as punch up to elbow. It's a simple movement that will increase your core strength so, so much. So when the workout calls for doing getups, just do punch up to elbows instead. Don't leave a hole in your workout. Substitute another exercise you can do.

STRENGTH SUMMARY

> Strength training is a skill to be mastered. If you treat it like that, you'll never get bored or burned out.

> Always value form over weight.

> Never train to failure (leave one or two in the tank).

> Kettlebells are a sport unto themselves that make you stronger and more athletic in real-life activities, not just sports or fitness.

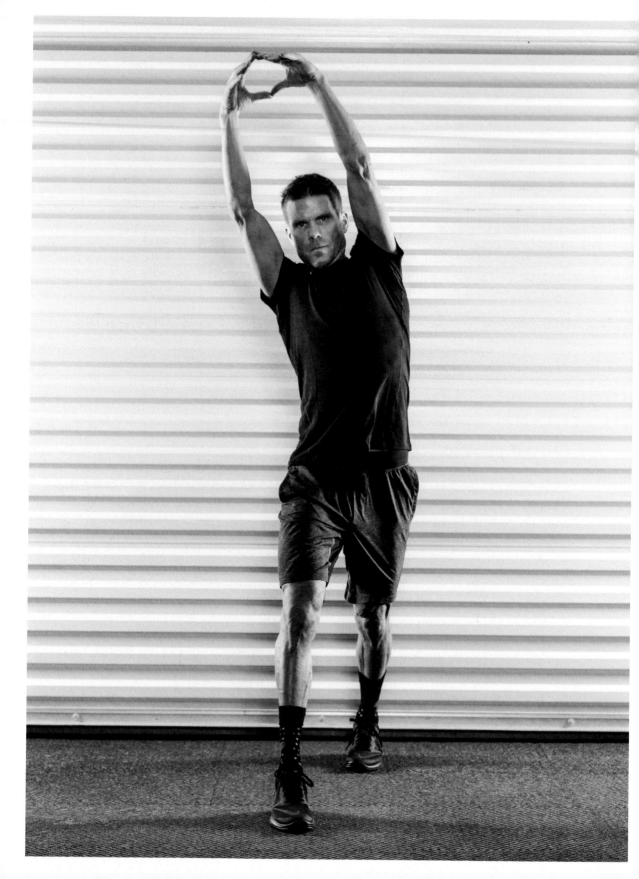

CHAPTER FIVE: RECOVERY

> ## Increasing Mobility Through Stretching, Self-Myofascial Massage, and Controlled Breathing

A BEAUTIFUL FRIENDSHIP
By Irving Azoff

Getting old sucks. Even worse: having to admit it to yourself. But I could deny it no longer. My knees and lower back were killing me, and I had to give up my beloved golf game. Then my friend Casey Wasserman hooked me up with Peter Park. "The guy's legit," Casey said. I'd see for myself. On the first day with Peter, he says to me, "Irving, let me see you touch your toes." So I say, "Peter, I've always been tight in that way, even when I was a kid, but it's never been an issue so—" But Peter says, "Do it anyway, Irving." So I try. I barely reached my knees. And that was just the beginning. Like the hard-ass he is, Peter puts me through more trials—which I also fail—and in summation he says, "Your T-spine is so congested that your weight distribution throughout your T-spine is gone. That means you'll take all of your load in your neck and lower spine. No way you could righteously swing a golf club in that condition. Also, your hamstrings are tight as piano strings, that's why you can't hinge or bend over without defaulting,"—back rounding, I later learned—"which is probably contributing to your lower back pain and causing your knee pain too. You're kind of a mess, Irving," he chuckles. Very funny. So I ask him how the hell I got to this sad state, and he says, "Sitting on your ass at work all day and old age and negligence and denial and—" "Piss off," I finally tell him. Peter just smiles. I ask him, "So what's next?" "Don't worry, Irving," he says. "You'll golf again. I promise." That was the beginning of our beautiful friendship.

I LOVE IRVING. OUR FRIENDSHIP IS built on a solid foundation of training and sarcasm. Irving is an inspiration. Not just because he's one of the most successful entertainment executives around, but also because despite his busy schedule, he never misses a workout; his training has become a ritual, and you don't mess with a ritual. His consistency is why he's made so many gains. (He can bend over without defaulting now and touch his palms flat on the floor.)

My friendship with Irving has begotten other friendships with clients Irving represents in the music business, like Harry Styles. For his age Harry's one of the wisest guys I know, has a great work ethic, and trains hard (sometimes too hard—I have to back him off), so he'll have a long career in a business known for flashes in the pan. A few years ago Harry insisted that there was someone I needed to meet, someone whose workout philosophies lined up perfectly with mine, a guy with magic hands. His name is Jussi Lomakka.

I'd already heard of Jussi but had never met the mythic soft-tissue specialist famous among fitness intelligentsia for his insight into why people might be in pain—and knowing just how to help them get out of it. The reason we never crossed paths was because he's so, so busy, constantly working and traveling to help his clients, including a long stint on the road with the band U2. But Harry made sure Jussi and I finally met, and it turns out that Harry-the-matchmaker was right. There truly was kismet from the start. One of the first things Jussi said to me (a perfect Jussi-ism, meaning short and right) was, "The best corrective exercise is doing the exercise correctly." Bingo.

Ever since, Jussi and I have been working together, sharing clients, with Jussi sending me people who need to learn how to move well again and get strong, and me sending Jussi my clients who are in pain or aren't recovering from injury, like my longtime client pro surfer Lakey Peterson. I've been training Lakey since she was a girl. Lakey's become so strong and fit over the years that she trains alongside my male pro athletes—and often puts them to shame. But Lakey broke her ankle surfing, and even after it healed, the joint stayed locked tight, and you can't surf at the competitive level without good ankle mobility, so she couldn't rejoin the tour. I tried everything I knew to help her and got so frustrated. So I connected her with Jussi, and in just two sessions Jussi got Lakey's ankle mobile again, and she returned to the tour. I also rely on Jussi's input on training, so his imprint is all over this book, though no more than in this chapter.

Regaining mobility through stretching and self-massage is the last of the five elements of your workout, but just because this chapter comes last doesn't mean it's the least important. In fact, if you're like Irving, you might get nowhere in your rebound without it.

As you grow older the sliding surfaces of your muscles get congested, and different depths of tissue get stuck together—they tighten and shorten. This is particularly true for those of us who sit at desks or in cars a lot (I'm the latter). We lose range of motion in the joints as a result, which affects how we walk, squat, stand—basically, it effects every movement we make. We become less mobile, in other words, incapable of going from one position to another with ease, thus putting limits on the activities we can do—or exposing ourselves to injury trying to do them. Tight, short muscles also are anathema to good posture.

By increasing your flexibility and releasing tight tissue, you'll increase your mobility, which means you'll move better, and that means you'll be capable of getting stronger and in better cardio shape. In other words, what you learn in this chapter might well be the catalyst to your rebound. A tall order? Hate stretching? Heard it's a waste of time? Or that foam rolling's so painful you don't even want to try it? Let me tell you a nightmare I suffered a few years ago and see if you change your mind.

I had some tendonitis in my right knee, so I went in for a routine cortisone shot and came out with a stubborn staph infection. My knee eventually required five operations to clean out, and I had to spend three hours every day in a hyperbaric chamber for oxygen therapy and for three months needed intravenous antibiotics. That was all followed by spending twelve weeks with my knee immobilized in a cast, which ended in disaster: X-rays showed that the muscles in my quad had calcified—they'd turned to bone. It was like something out of a horror movie. I couldn't bend my knee anymore. My doctor put me under three times to "break open" the joint (hell yeah, it hurt) and then told me that due to scar tissue and shortened muscles, I'd never get back the last 30 to 40 percent range of motion (ROM). Which meant I'd never run, ski, cycle, or do a thousand other things again. I would limp through the rest of my life. I can't tell you how pissed off I was. I didn't do anything wrong—this wasn't my fault! But one thing was for sure: I did not accept that prognosis.

ROM matters because without full flexion (bending of knee) or terminal extension (straightening your leg), your body alters its gait pattern: you walk and move inefficiently as your body compensates for the injury any way it can, which can cause problems to your hips, knees, ankles, and lower back. Also, without terminal extension, your quads can't contract and simply won't fire, so they grow weaker, creating imbalances that cause even more problems such as a tilted pelvis and lower back pain. There are no simple answers to regaining lost ROM. No doctor can surgically get it back for you. The only method I knew of was good old-fashioned persistence. That meant stretching everyday to get my muscle surfaces sliding better and the muscles in the quad lengthened again. Once the sliding surfaces of the muscles are restored, the tissue would lengthen and become more pliable. And foam rolling and smashing on a hard softball would break up scar tissue around the injury and would help loosen tightened tissue.

There are many kinds of stretching, such as static stretching (those long holds you did before football or softball practice back in high school). I'm not a fan. There's ballistic stretching, a pulsing forward and backward into and out of the stretch, which I do during certain stretches like pigeon. But the stretching Jussi and I have gotten the most success from—for ourselves and our clients—has been active-passive stretching (APS).

The theory behind active-passive stretching is actually kind of cool. During a stretch, when you reach your endpoint (you can stretch no further without feeling as if the muscle will tear), you do a five-second contraction (provide resistance against the stretch), then release the contraction and quickly go deeper into the stretch. By doing that, you've taken advantage of a split-second in time when you can go deeper into the stretch without tearing the muscle. So contract the muscle, then let it out and go deeper into the stretch. Active-passive stretching practiced over time improves the sliding surfaces of your tissue, the mobility of the muscle, and the joint range of motion. And you can do active-passive stretching on your own, which is key.

And I did do it on my own—a lot. I did many different stretches for my whole body, but I focused on two that my knee needed most, *couch stretch* for my quads and *pigeon stretch* for my hips. When I first started, my quad was so tight and the scar tissue so built up that I couldn't even get into position. I had a long road ahead. *Pigeon stretch* is tough even when you don't have an injury. With your knee bent at 90 degrees in front and beneath you and your other leg extended behind you, you hinge forward, trying to bring your chest to your knee without rounding your back. When I tried it, I nearly tipped over. A long journey indeed.

And that journey would have to include breaking down the scar tissue that had built up in my knee. That meant rolling out all four muscles of my tight quads on a foam roller and smashing my hamstrings and glutes on a hard softball because my tissue had seized up from inactivity. I'd lost pliability and was rigid like a board.

During that time I still trained, doing upper-body weights and cardio on the Concept 2 SkiErg (there's never an excuse—you can always find a way to train). After every workout I took advantage of my body being warmed up, stretching and rolling and smashing. I also incorporated controlled breathing, because when you breathe you let go of tension and go deeper into your muscles and tissue. An unexpected benefit was that controlled breathing also focused me at the end of training, put me in a meditative state, and helped me let go of my frustrations and anger. I probably needed that as much as anything!

It took nearly a year before the scar tissue in my knee broke up and my quad and hips reopened. I finally got back most of my mobility and range of motion. That meant I could start running, biking, skiing—and doing a thousand other things again. And if you, dear reader, have limitations, as I did, with persistence and what you learn in the following pages you can overcome some or all of yours too.

During the four weeks of movement practice you're going to learn twelve stretches and smashes for the anterior (front of body) and posterior (back of body) parts of your body. Each stretch and smash takes two to four minutes, so your goal will be to learn which stretch and smash you need most and incorporate them into your workouts. But be consistent and persistent, or you're wasting your time. And it's not recommended to do recovery work before training. Mobilizing the joints before a workout destabilizes them, opening you up to injury.

SO WHAT'S WRONG WITH YOU?

If you have specific issues, aches, and pains (not tears and breaks!) and you want to focus on specific muscles or joints at home or during Recovery practice, by all means do it. But you might need some guidance. The body is a complicated and interconnected piece of physiology, so the path to alleviating pain is not always as straightforward as simply attacking what hurts. The following are some examples that might guide you to solutions for your aches and pains.

ANKLES

After March Madness ends for college basketball, April Crazy begins for me. Because that's when the NBA draft picks start to prepare for tryouts and combines where they show off their skills, strengths, and athletic ability to the scouts and coaches who might draft them. It's their audition. Every year sports agent Casey Wasserman sends me a lot of these young, talented athletes to get them ready. And as I do with all new clients, I first watch how they move. Despite their youth, a lot of them have pain and injuries and don't move right, and I have to figure out why—and fix them. Scouts and coaches can smell injury and dysfunction a mile away, so the players have to move well on the court.

With basketball players I always start with their ankles. Why? Ankles are ground zero: they take on the body's full weight during jumping and running. And basketball players run and jump a lot—and sprain and twist and tear their ankles. Ankles are meant to be a mobile joint (as opposed to the knee, a stable joint), and when they tighten up, they lose mobility, and that sometimes trickles upward and destabilizes the knees. You'd be surprised how many people, not just basketball players, I see with tight ankles that are the cause of knee pain.

Immobile ankles also can cause faulty squat patterns. The ankle becomes too immobile to get low, the heels rise off the floor, and the back rounds and defaults. Not only can that lead to lower back pain and inhibit development of core and glute strength, but it also means that basketball players can't get into a proper defensive position, good and low with a flat back, out of which they can explode. Tight ankles can also affect the Achilles and the calf muscles, which pull and tear easily.

The Recovery solution (you'll find all these detailed in the following chapters):

- ankle mobility exercises

- couch stretch

- calf and shin smash

- hamstring stretch

- hamstring smash

KNEES

Think of your knees like this: their role is to connect the lower leg (fibula and tibia) to the upper leg (femur), the knee becoming a sort of mediator between them. Therefore, if something's going wrong down below, such as in the ankles, the knees might be the canary in the coal mine, so to speak, an indication that something's wrong. And you should listen. And it works both directions. If the hip complex and the tissue surrounding the pelvis are compromised (tight), your knees or lower spine will let you know. Listen to your knees.

If you don't know the source of your knee pain, I recommend you do a lot of different stretches and tissue work to make sure you're covering all bases. As I just said, poor ankle mobility can cause instability and therefore pain in the knees. When quads get tight, they wreak havoc on knee stability because the four quadriceps along with the hamstrings are the knees' main stabilizers and can draw the kneecap out of alignment, which causes tracking problems. And if you have glute amnesia, well, weak glutes are often the cause of knee pain, so you know you have to stretch the hip flexors and smash and strengthen your glutes.

> ### > THE RECOVERY SOLUTION:

- quad roll

- ankle mobility

- glute/TFL smash

- pigeon on bench

- calf smash

QUADS

I already said that quad tightness can cause knee pain. But so can overly developed quads and underdeveloped hamstrings and glutes. Such imbalances can cause glute amnesia and lower back pain. Some runners have quads so tight that their gait's thrown off, their performance sags, or they get injured.

> THE RECOVERY SOLUTION:

- couch stretch

- quad roll

- hamstring and glute/TFL smash

- psoas smash or diaphragm smash

HIPS

One day I was working with a group of NBA prospects, all centers and forwards, when Jerry West came into the gym. He told me that the problem that big guys in the league have is that very few of them can get low and into an athletic position and take up space in and around the key. What he was saying, in other words, is they lack the mobility to cover ground and play as big as they are. I've found that most of those guys have tight ankles and hips, which causes hip immobility and tightened tissue, and that leads to faulty movement patterns and, over the years, injury.

The other leading cause of tight hips, as I said earlier, is chronic sitting. I come across very few who sit a lot whose hips haven't gotten tight over time.

> THE RECOVERY SOLUTION:

- pigeon stretch on bench

- glute/TFL smash

- hamstring stretch

- hamstring smash

HAMSTRINGS

Tight hamstrings keep you from hinging or bending over without defaulting (rounding your back). That can cause your glutes to shut off, weaken, and stop supporting your lower back. Pain ensues. Tight hamstrings can also keep you from getting into efficient athletic positions without defaulting. Cyclists sometimes can't get into a low, aerodynamic position; runners' strides shorten; and golfers can't hinge well for full range of motion driving and effective putting.

> THE RECOVERY SOLUTION:

- hamstring stretch

- hamstring smash

- glute/TFL smash

- psoas or diaphragm smash

LOWER BACK

Lower back pain is practically an epidemic these days and why Dr. Eric Goodman and I created Foundation training. As I've written already, a lot of lower back pain comes from chronic sitting and inactivity, which leads to bad posture, imbalances, weak glutes, and no support for the lower back. The Foundation exercises you're going to do in the Movement chapter will benefit you greatly. But during Recovery you can smash and roll to assist in overcoming pain.

> THE RECOVERY SOLUTION:

- psoas or diaphragm smash

- glute/TFL smash

- T-spine smash

- couch stretch

THORACIC SPINE (T-SPINE)

Irving Azoff couldn't swing a golf club because his T-spine was so congested and his mid- to upper back didn't have the mobility anymore to rotate as needed to properly perform a golf swing. When that happened, a lot of the rotation shifted to his lower back, and pain ensued. It also inhibited his shoulder mobility. Golfers, baseball players, and any athlete who needs good rotation from the spine need to work on opening up the T-spine.

> THE RECOVERY SOLUTION:

- T-spine rotations

- T-spine smash

- glute/TFL smash

- psoas smash

- lat-to-rotator cuff roll

SHOULDERS

Chronic sitting can also take the brunt of the blame for shoulder problems. So many of us these days sit all day at a keyboard, our shoulders slumped forward, inch-by-inch ruining our posture. That causes lower back pain, shoulder immobility, and T-spine immobility. You can't effectively roll or smash your shoulders, but you can get into the areas around them to help loosen up the tissue. By doing the following exercises you'll open up your overhead shoulder position, which is key for good posture and healthy shoulder mechanics.

> THE RECOVERY SOLUTION:

- pec smash

- lat-to-rotator cuff roll

- T-spine smash

- T-spine rotations

QUESTION: How often should I do my Recovery routine?

ANSWER: You'll do one stretch and one smash or roll after every workout. However, you can stretch, roll, and smash as much as you like at home. I usually end my day stretching and smashing while watching sports on TV.

QUESTION: How long do I do each stretch, roll, and smash?

ANSWER: Unfortunately it's hard to say how long it will take to make headway during Recovery. Everyone's different, and it will depend on your tolerance for pain. I tell my clients to stretch, roll, and smash until they feel an effective change. I know that's imprecise, so if you need something more concrete, during your Recovery routine go for at least two minutes for each stretch, roll, or smash.

QUESTION: I'm still not clear what exactly smashing is?

ANSWER: You are trying to improve muscle surfaces for more efficient sliding in between different depths of the tissue. Smashing your myofascial tissue typically is done with a hard softball, baseball, lacrosse ball, peanut ball (two balls connected, just stick them in a sock). Because balls are round (newsflash, right?), you can roll your tissue over them, "smashing" it, so to speak. You simply roll your body over the designated spot, using body weight to apply pressure. Sometimes you'll move in a circular pattern, searching for sticky spots that need extra attention. Other times you'll smash in a windshield-wiper or smearing motion as you move up and down the muscle. I give you the cues you need to effectively smash.

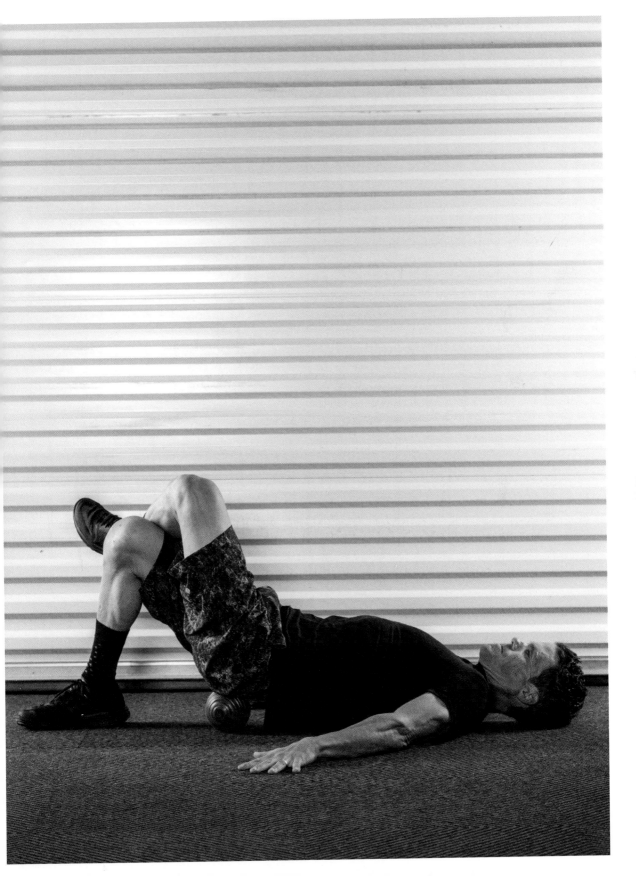

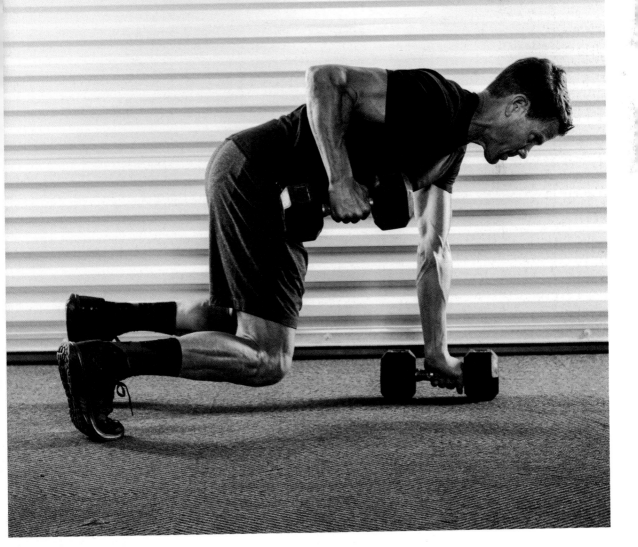

PART TWO
HOW TO TRAIN THE REBOUND WAY
> TENSIONING FOR STRENGTH AND MOVEMENT PRACTICE

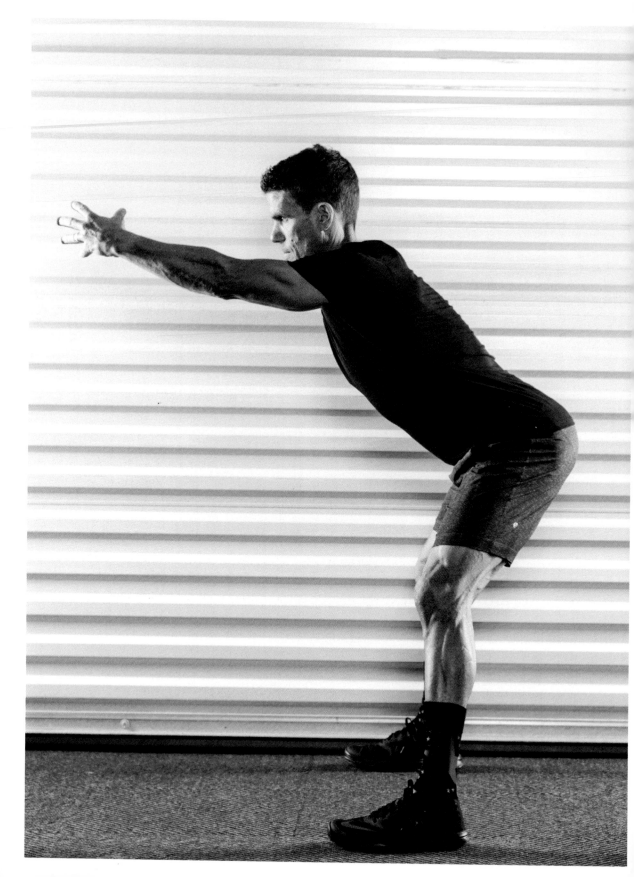

CHAPTER SIX: TENSIONING FOR STRENGTH

A WHOLE CHAPTER ON TENSION? Like you don't already have enough of *that* in your life. Well, this is a different kind of tension. The good kind of tension you create during exercise to make you stronger and keep you safe. Never heard of tensioning? Neither had my good friend "Wesley."

Wesley used to be a terrific athlete. He played college football and later became obsessed with golf. And he was *good*. Unfortunately, because of chronic lower back pain, he couldn't play anymore. It just hurt him too damn much. But he loved the sport and was willing to do anything to get back on the links. He tried chiropractors, had back surgery, took painkillers, but nothing helped him. I met Wesley almost by chance. He was vacationing in Santa Barbara and threw his back totally out of whack. A doctor we both know asked if I could help him out. When Wesley got to Platinum he could barely move or stand up. His back was in acute spasm. I had Wesley walk and move, and I could see the snowball effect that had occurred over the years. He'd stopped training, his body weakened, especially his posterior chain, his T-spine had stiffened, his movement patterns deteriorated, and pain was the outcome. I told Wesley he'd have to learn to move all over again and then rebuild his strength if he ever wanted to get out of pain. He did, he was desperate, so he changed his vacation plans extending his stay in Santa Barbara so we could work together. During the first few sessions I had to teach him piece-by-piece how to move again. We started slowly with shallow, elementary Foundation exercises, and what I noticed about Wesley was that he didn't just move with bad patterns, but he was also sloppy, loose, and slack. He had no *tension* in his body.

So what exactly is tension as it relates to the body and to exercise? I first learned about the concept of creating tension when I was a nineteen year old, working out with some of the strongest powerlifters around. They taught me that when you create tension throughout your body before an exercise and hold onto it during, it prepares your body to brace for the movement, it increases your performance, and makes you safer. And when I worked with Pavel, he taught me that proper tensioning made you 20 to 30 percent stronger during exercise. But when Eric Goodman and I created Foundation Training to help people break free from back pain, that's when I really learned how important tensioning is, especially when it comes to moving well and recovering from injury. Back to Wesley.

As I said, Wesley had never heard of tensioning as it relates to exercise, so I had to teach him. I started with a Founder, a pose you'll learn very soon. I had Wesley stand with his feet shoulder-width apart and begin corkscrewing (anchoring) his feet into the floor to create lower-body tension. Then he squeezed his glutes tightly and braced his abs as if he's about to take a punch. Wesley could really feel the tension he was creating, and was surprised he could get into the pose. But as soon as he let go of the tension and went slack again, the supporting muscles surrounding his lower back turned back off and pain shot through his back. Wesley had a long way to go. What about you? Let's give it a try?

Like Wesley, stand upright with your feet shoulder-width apart. Now, keeping your feet anchored, try to corkscrew them into the floor (right foot tries to turn clockwise, left counterclockwise). You should feel tension all the way up through your legs to your glutes. Now squeeze your glutes together. Lastly sniff in a shallow breath of air, and brace your abs like you're about to get punched in the gut. No part of your body should move. But almost every part should be tensed. If so, congratulations! You're creating tension.

Okay, now you can relax! Whether you're about to do an exercise or pick up your kid, if you create tension first and hold onto it during the movement, the body anticipates and prepares to take on the weight and uses all the tensed muscles to help execute it, including, as you just learned, the legs, glutes, abs and core, but also the chest, shoulders and arms, and a ton of little muscles you don't even realize you have. The exercise becomes a team effort. And soon creating tension during your workout becomes habit outside in the real world. You'll create tension as you hinge over to pick up dirty laundry, squat down to lift a dumbbell at the gym, or as you pick tomatoes or beans in your garden. It will become second nature. Conversely, if you don't learn to create tension during exercise and your body isn't prepared to take on the weight, you might get loose and sloppy, just like Wesley, and most of the lifting will fall to the fulcrum that is your lower back. That will lead to problems.

Wesley had no strength in his lower back, hips, and glutes—in other words, his whole posterior chain was shutting down. During his stay in Santa Barbara, we worked two hours a day as Wesley learned how to move right again, incorporating tension into every move he made. And Wesley made a lot of progress, but finally after three weeks, he had to go home to his family and his job.

Wesley's a busy man and I was worried that he'd stop practicing his movements and would relapse back into pain, so we FaceTime trained four days a week. As time went by, creating tension became second nature, he added a little weight to some of the movements, and he got stronger and his pain diminished. Within six to eight weeks he was doing full-range squats. That was huge!

After about six months, Wesley was back playing golf again. He was so happy. It had been three years since he'd played. But he's not all the way out of the woods yet. Sometimes Wesley still gets busy and stressed, doesn't put in the maintenance work, he starts to get loose and sloppy again, and his back issues pop back up as a reminder of what he needs to do. The beautiful thing is that now he has the tools to get back to his movement practice and get himself out of pain. Corkscrewing, glute squeezing, and ab bracing are just a few of the many kinds of tensioning you need to learn. You'll also need to learn techniques that go along with creating tension like proper exercise breathing. In fact, let's start there.

BREATHING

The technique of breathing during exercise confuses a lot of people. Should I inhale down and exhale up? Do I hold my breath or breathe in and out really fast? Here's a quick and easy way to think about breathing during exercise. Most exercises (at least the ones in this book) have two parts. For instance, with pushups you lower yourself down (part 1) and then push yourself back up (part 2). During squats you lower yourself down and then power yourself back up. Right? Eccentric movements are the down half and, you may've noticed, are typically the easier part of the exercise. So think of taking that sniff of air (eccentric) as preparation for the harder part, part two, the *concentric movement*, for which you'll emit a quick, short burst of air for power. For instance, before you squat down (eccentric) take in a sniff of air, then lower your body toward the floor. As you're rising up (concentric) you let out the air near the top of the squat to help power you up. Sniff in to prepare, let out for power.

Why a sniff of air? I say sniff because I want you to take a breath in through your nose because it will help you brace your abs. The two are connected. (Try it—sniff in fast but controlled.) And the let out with a "tttssss." (Put your tongue on your upper palate, letting out a short, fast "Tttssss!" sound, like a hissing snake.) The "tttssss" out is a way of controlling how much air you let out. If you let out too much, you get too loose. If you let out just the right amount of air, you'll maintain tension. So sniff in for control, breathe out for power. Sniff in air eccentric, breathe out concentric. You might get a few funny looks at the gym, but just ignore those folks—you certainly don't need any more of *that* kind of tension in your life.

CREATING TENSION THROUGHOUT THE BODY

CORKSCREWING FEET

Corkscrewing your feet into the floor activates the lower body, stabilizes the pelvis, and makes movements such as squats and deadlifts safer and more powerful. Before you begin such movements you'll grip the floor with your feet and try to screw them into the ground—left foot tries to turn counter-clockwise, right attempts clockwise rotation—though of course your feet don't actually move at all. That's what creates the tension in your lower body that activates your glutes and hamstrings, the lower back's chief supporters, and prepares them to take on the weight.

What to focus on when corkscrewing your feet:

- Stay on your midfoot.

- Grip the floor with your toes.

- Visualize screwing your feet into the floor to create tension.

CORKSCREWING HANDS

Corkscrewing your hands during pushups or a plank brings in your lat muscles and packs down your shoulders, making any upper-body exercise stronger, safer, and more effective. Corkscrewing hands also puts your shoulders in a much stronger and safer position. Before you begin any movement in plank position, grip the floor firmly with your palms, then try to screw your hands in to the floor—left hand tries to turn counter-clockwise, right goes clockwise. As you corkscrew, you'll feel your shoulders pack down and your lats activate or turn on. Squeeze your heels and glutes together, brace your abs, and take in a sniff of air. Now you're ready to do a pushup, hold a plank, or row a dumbbell.

GLUTE SQUEEZE

Every Foundation movement, exercise, and even many stretches I teach require creating tension in the glutes. Glute squeezes help stabilize the pelvis and put your back in a stronger, safer neutral position. Even doing a glute squeeze during pushups creates tension and draws the core into the movement. And the glute squeeze is so simple to execute that you don't even need any cues. Just breathe and squeeze your buns together.

SCISSOR TENSION

By "scissoring" your feet and legs in a lunging position (one foot forward, one back), you create full lower-body tension for lunge stretches, knee drops, and other movements. To create scissor tension, stand in a split stance or lunge position, then pull the front foot backward (without actually moving it), and pull the back foot forward (without moving) at the same time. You'll feel your legs and glutes tense up and your pelvis stabilize.

AB BRACING

Ab bracing is all about preparedness. It makes the core instantly more stable and, in many exercises, works alongside the glutes to protect the lower back by taking the brunt of the heavy lifting. Before bracing your abs always sniff in a breath of air, then tighten your abs as if you're about to take a punch in the gut. Then you're ready to initiate the exercise.

LAT LOCKING

Locking down your lats—the latissimus dorsi muscles of your back and sides—keeps your shoulders from shrugging up during many exercises such as pushups, rows, and dead lifts. When you drop or pack your shoulders down and lock your lats tight, you create stability in every movement—and also improve your posture by flattening your back. Lat locking is particularly important in cycling. I see so many people who ride with their shoulders shrugged up around their ears in such a terrible postural position! Lock in those lats, and your shoulders will shrug down with them. To lock your lats, put your arms at your sides, turn your thumbs pointing outward, pull your shoulders back and down. Locking your lats instantly straightens your posture.

SPHERE OF TENSION

The sphere of tension. Sounds like the next Indiana Jones flick, right? It's not quite that adventurous, perhaps, but the sphere of tension is a key technique that draws in the core and the upper body during Foundation movements, such as the founder. So as you corkscrew your feet, squeeze your glutes, brace your abs, and lock your lats, creating a sphere of tension—that final step—means now your whole body is engaged.

Try creating a sphere of tension by extending your arms out in front of you and putting your fingertips together like you're forming a sphere (see photo). Now push your fingers against each other to create tension, take a sniff of air, and brace your abs—you'll feel your pecs and shoulders tense up too. (Don't let your shoulders shrug up.) This means most of your upper body is turned on.

QUESTION: I've been training in gyms for years, I weigh the same, I haven't gotten any stronger. Is that because I'm not creating tension?

ANSWER: There could be a lot of reasons: Tensioning, boredom with the same, old routine, poor training techniques, but this book is designed to overcome those issues, so if those are your problems, problem solved. One obstacle a lot of people have is a poor training mindset or a lack of clear purpose in the gym, and for that I'll give you a tip from the pros. The great athletes like Justin Verlander, Diana Taurasi, Lance Armstrong step into the gym and instantly become what I call, "Terminatorized." Almost like actors taking the stage, they transform and become single-minded in purpose—and that purpose ain't to socialize. Once they get their head in the game, the outside world disappears and they focus on every circuit, exercise, rep, every pedal of the bike, stroke on the SkiErg, stride on the treadmill, trying to get the most out of them. You won't always feel like you can kick ass, not every day, even pro athletes don't, but you can go as hard as possible on that particular day and if you do that, you've still won. And that's how you make progress.

THE OCCUPATIONAL ATHLETE: A RECIPE FOR STAYING ON THE JOB
By Kelly Park

To all the chefs and waiters, construction workers and gardeners, doctors and nurses, grocery store cashiers and stockers, dog groomers and policemen who rely on your physical health to do your jobs: I know how hard it is to work on your feet all day, come home, ass kicked, and you just want to plop down in front of the tube, have a glass of wine, and chill the rest of the night. Especially because your back or your knee hurts (which is why you've been taking so much ibuprofen lately). But your job isn't just work, is it? It's what you do. It's who you are. And it's how you make your living. You want to excel at it and have longevity. But as you get older, I know firsthand that to have the strength and stamina to function at the top of your game, you have to train for your job as if your livelihood depends on it. Because it does.

I know the thought of going to the gym before or after work sounds impossible. Believe me, I know. I've been an acute care nurse for twenty-two years. I'm on my feet sometimes working thirteen-hour shifts—I squat down, hinge over, lift two-hundred-pound patients all day long, and, at forty-seven, I don't recover like I used to. To keep up, I have to make the time to train at least three times a week.

It's not easy, I know, so I typically go to the gym on my days off. I treat those workouts almost like "spa days," doing a lot of stretching and mobility work but also strength training and cardio to relieve stress. And it works. I still have the stamina to do those long shifts, my energy levels stay high throughout, and I'm focused, efficient, and better at my job—all because I keep fit. I want to keep working as long as I can.

In addition to being a full-time nurse, I own Platinum Fitness with my husband, Peter Park. As a gym owner, trainer, and a nurse, I have some tips that might help you, especially if you just don't have the time to get to the gym.

Do the Movement Practice workouts regularly, and they will change how you move on the job. As we age, our movement patterns deteriorate, so every time you lift a box, a sofa, or a human being you're reinforcing bad patterns and heading for the disability line. Learning how to move right again will help you avoid injury, get out of pain, and do your job more efficiently.

Strength. You need to be strong to work. If going to the gym isn't possible, buy two kettlebells and do Peter's Rebound workouts at home. Kettlebells aren't expensive, they take up virtually no room, and if you have two (one lighter, one heavier), you can do most of the workouts in this book. Staying strong is key to overcoming and preventing injury and to career longevity.

Cardio. Your heart's important, and cardio is a big stress reliever. So make time to do some cardio training. Even if you just take a twenty-minute walk after work to wind down and get rid of stress, it will help. And trust me: as a nurse who's seen it all, taking a walk is a lot healthier than drinking alcohol or taking prescription drugs to relieve stress. Good luck!

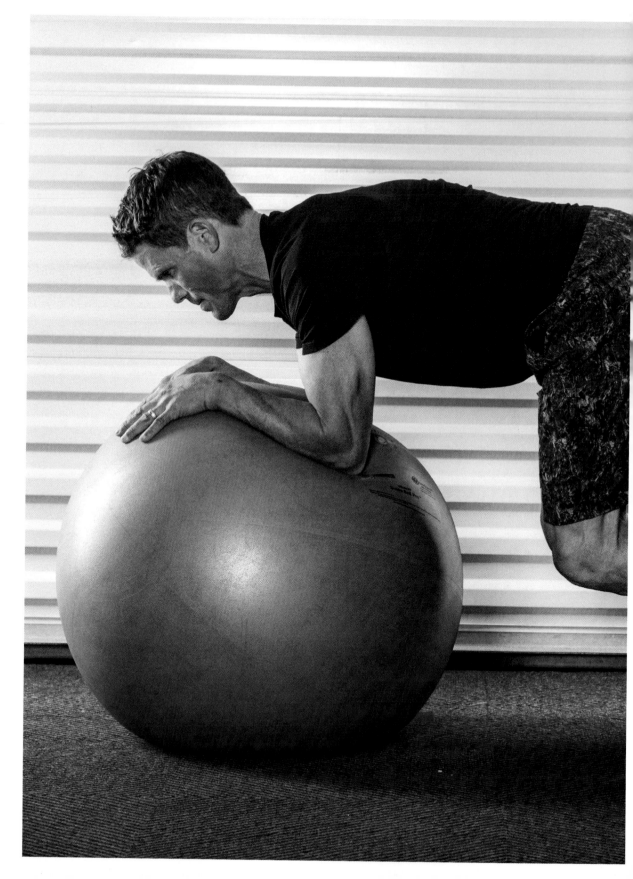

CHAPTER SEVEN: MOVEMENT PRACTICE

ED SNIDER WAS ONE OF MY first clients, a true mentor and inspiration, and he became a close friend. A successful entrepreneur (he owned the Philadelphia 76ers and the Flyers hockey team), smart, tough, and generous, for twenty-six years we trained, sweated, huffed, and puffed together. Ed was strong as an ox. Even in his eighties he had perfect, stick-straight posture and moved more like a thirty-year-old. I thought for sure Ed would outlive me! But then he got bladder cancer. Still, Ed refused to give up—he was going to beat his disease. We kept training together three, four, five days a week, mostly doing movement practice, the fundamental, unloaded exercises that build and maintain good movement patterns. And although there's no way to know if our training together prolonged Ed's life, I do know they improved the time he had left. In the end Ed didn't leave anything on the table. And he always lived as he moved—with grace. Go get 'em, Ed!

MOVEMENT PRACTICE

Time to get your body moving well again. For the next four weeks you'll retrain your faulty patterns, start eating a healthy-fats diet, and begin doing low-intensity, base-building cardiovascular exercise—and do some Recovery work as well. Although you can practice the movements in this chapter at home or in your office, now's the time to start making your training into a ritual, one that you refuse to miss. For most of us that probably means going to the gym.

Let's start with a few tips on how to start eating a healthy fats diet.

HEALTHY FATS

As I mention in Chapter One, the best way for you to control what you eat is to shop for and prepare your own food. When you go out and buy real foods again—organic chickens and vegetables, grass-fed beef and bison, wild caught fish—you start to fall in love with your food. To get you started, here are a few tips from me and my wife, Kelly.

- Shop at your farmer's market where all the vegetables, eggs, and meats are grown locally by people you may even know. Everything at the farmer's market is typically fresher than what you get at the supermarket. That means it tastes better, for sure, but also it will keep longer. That's a big time-saver, because you can stock up and don't have to go shopping as often.

- Remember to cook food ahead of time so you have it on hand. You're less likely to go carb-diving (fall off the wagon) if you have sautéed broccoli and wild-caught salmon sitting ready to eat in the fridge. Some of my favorite vegetables to cook ahead and reheat are onions, mushrooms, kale, broccoli, cauliflower, and, within limits, sweet potatoes.

- Always keep the ingredients for a salad on hand. A salad can mean almost anything, but try a bunch of thrice-washed spinach, arugula, avocado, cooked beets, tomatoes, and cucumbers when they're in season or hard-boiled egg. And then toss on leftover protein like chicken breast, sliced steak, or fish—even canned tuna and salmon works well.

- Buy raw almonds and macadamia nuts and roast them (375 degrees for about ten minutes, giving the pan a shake every three or so minutes), and keep them around as snacks. (Careful how many you eat: they're fat-rich, which is why we like them, but a small handful will do.)

- One of my favorite foods is a baked whole chicken. You can buy them already cooked in most grocery stores, but try baking one yourself—it's easier than pie. (Rinse, pat dry, salt, then bake breast side up in a shallow pan with chunks of onion, carrot, parsnips, fennel at 450 degrees for about an hour or until the breast is 160 degrees.) A whole chicken is the gift that keeps on giving: dinner, leftovers for breakfast, salads, lunch the next day—you can even make chicken stock with the bones for soup or to enrich your vegetable stir-fries.

That's a good start, filling your diet with good, healthy-fat foods. And by doing so, you've filled in the gap left by all that carb cutting you're doing.

It's also time to cut down on sugar intake. Start with your morning coffee. The good news is the quality of coffee has gotten so high that you don't want to put sugar in it—that only masks the incredible deep flavors going on inside your cup. But feel free to add a tad of half-and-half or whole cream to it. (Half-and-half has just one gram of sugar and cream has none.)

Enough nutrition tips for now. Time to start moving. Below I describe all the basic movements you'll learn over the next four weeks. You can practice the movements individually, but it's important to learn them in the order of the circuit sequences I've laid out. Don't rush through the circuits. Treat each rep and exercise individually.

As for the cardio workouts, my directions are short and to the point for a reason. The goal here is simply to start base building and learn how to find your MAHR. Learning to do those things will take time. I also recommend you start doing a long cardio workout on the weekends. Cycle, hike, walk, jog—just get outside, if weather permits, and enjoy yourself.

ACTIVATION

> ANKLE MOBILITY

Poor ankle mobility is sometimes the underlying reason people have knee or hip problems. In fact, the first thing I look at when I see poor squatting mechanics is ankle mobility. So before every workout we're going to work on getting your ankles mobile again.

You're going to do it in a standing position. Start by leaning with your palms against a wall, and put one foot behind you and one in front of you. Bend the front knee, and drive it over the toe as far as you can without the heel coming up. Pulse ten times while driving your knee outward. You're flexing, or as we sometimes call it, flossing your ankle back and forth.

Now do ten more pulses driving your knee toward the middle, then ten more driving your knee inward. Then switch to your other ankle and repeat.

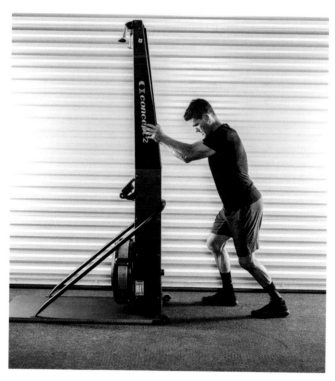

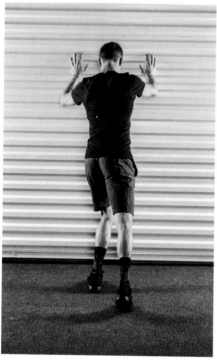
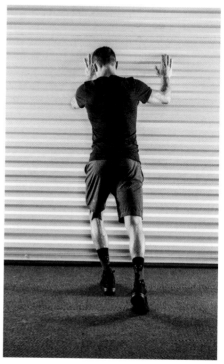

> BIRD DOGS

When a hunting dog locates a fallen bird, it stops, stiffens its body (creating tension), and points itself toward the bird for the hunter to find. When doing bird dogs, you won't be pointing at any dead birds, but you will be down on all fours like a dog, lifting opposing arms and legs, creating instability, which forces you to stabilize or tip over. Choose the former.

Begin on all fours, hands directly underneath your shoulders, hips and knees at 90 degrees. Tuck your pelvis forward, pulling your ribs down to flatten your back so your spine remains neutral. Your head should be facing straight down to the floor with your chin pulled back. Start creating tension by corkscrewing both hands into the ground. Take in a sniff of air, and brace your core.

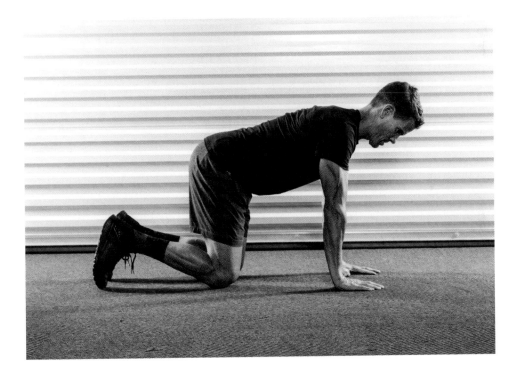

Now you'll do two things at once. Reach your right arm out, turning your right thumb away from you, and at the same time lift and lengthen your left (opposite) leg until both limbs are fully extended. Now squeeze your left glute tightly. Make sure your back stays in neutral position, pelvis tucked, and your hips stay square to the floor (don't let them tilt to one side). Hold this position for two seconds, then return to starting position and alternate with the other side.

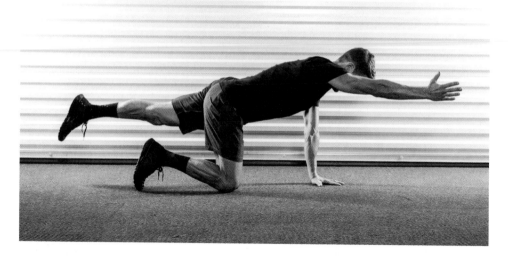

> T-SPINE ROTATIONS

The T-spine, or *thoracic spine*, are the twelve vertebrae starting from your midback and extending up toward the neck. If you sit a lot, the T-spine can become locked or immobile, and that can lead to shoulder, neck, and lower back problems. In a perfect world all my clients' T-spines would be mobile and their lumbar spines stable. A mobile T-spine is essential for all humans, but it's a must for people involved in sports like baseball and golf that require great thoracic rotation to swing safely and effectively. I like to activate the T-spine at the start of every workout to correct that negative pattern.

For the sake of efficiency, you'll always do T-spine rotations after bird dogs because they both have the same starting position. So as with bird dogs, start on all fours, with your hands directly underneath your shoulders and your hips and knees at 90 degrees. Put your right hand behind your head. To begin, reach your right elbow to your left elbow.

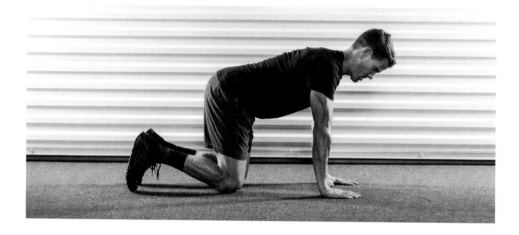

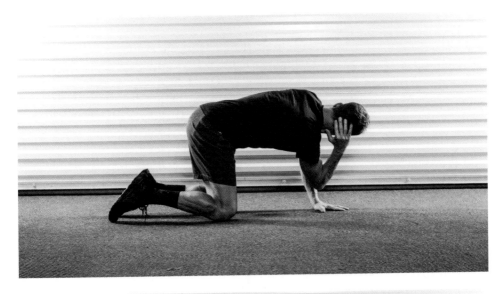

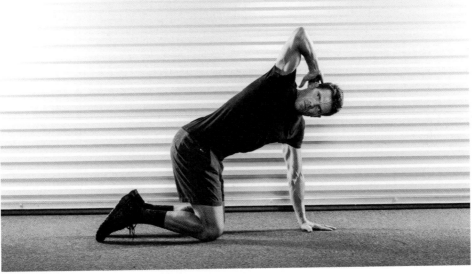

Now slowly rotate your right side upward, elbow leading the way, twisting up as far as possible while keeping your hips square. Focus on pulling from your upper spine and lats. Then slowly return to the starting position. When finished switch sides.

> EIGHT-POINT PLANK

Two hands, two elbows, two knees, and two toes—those are the eight points of a proper eight-point plank. Eight-point plank stiffens the core and develops good core strength and stability, but I also love eight-point planks because they teach you how to create tension practically from nothing. One warning: if it feels like nothing's happening, that's because you're not working hard enough. You really have to pull hard from all eight points for these planks to be effective.

Start in the bird dog position, with your hands directly underneath you and knees on the ground. Now dig your toes into the floor, and drop down so your elbows and forearms are directly below or slightly ahead of your shoulders on the floor, and pull your hips forward and tuck your pelvis, making sure your spine is neutral and hips are square to the floor. (You might need to watch yourself in a mirror to make sure you're in the correct position.) Now, dig all eight points into the floor—toes, knees, elbows, fingers—and pull tension to your core and hold it.

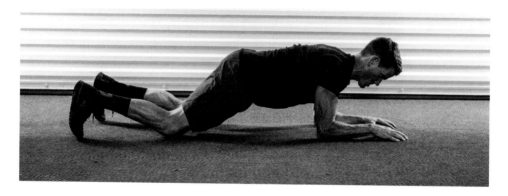

In the eight-point plank variation below, you lift your knees two inches off the ground. You'll be surprised how much this small change challenges your core and stability.

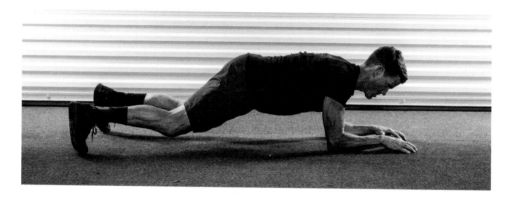

> FOUNDER

The founder is a simple yet powerful pose that strengthens your posterior chain and core, and it teaches you how to create full-body tension. The founder is the centerpiece of the Foundation program and emphasizes strong posture and acts as a building block for many other exercises in the coming workouts.

Begin by standing with your feet shoulder-width apart. Corkscrew your feet into the floor to create tension. Make sure your knees are back, almost straight. Now squeeze your glutes. Take a sniff of air, and brace your abs as if preparing to take a gut punch.

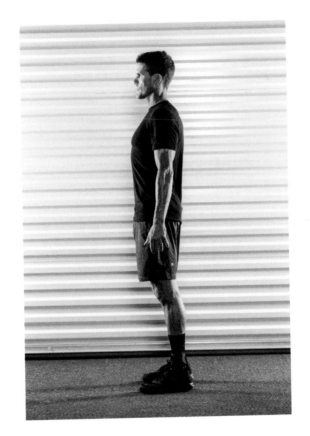

Slowly hinge your hips back as if pushing a drawer closed with your butt, chest hinging forward, equal and opposite to your hips. Make sure your ribs stay down and back stays flat and that your knees are still pushed back so they're nearly but not quite straight. Bring your extended arms behind you. Turn your thumbs away from you, pointing outward. Pull your shoulders down, and lock your lats.

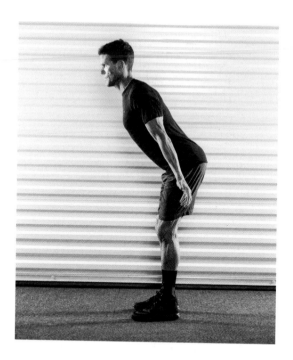

Now, reach out in front of you, extending your arms to shoulder height, and create a sphere of tension, and actively pull your shoulders back (no shrugging allowed). Your whole body should be engaged in the act of tensioning at this point.

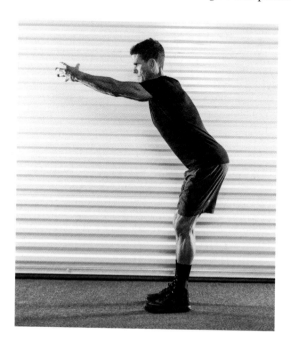

> WIDE FOUNDER

The *wide founder* notches things up another level from founder, bringing your adductors, those small muscles of your groin that get tight and shorten up, into play.

Start with your feet in a wide stance, feet corkscrewed into the floor pointed straight ahead, glutes squeezed. Take a sniff of air through your nose, brace your core, then slowly hinge your hips back while your chest moves forward, equal and opposite. Make sure your spine stays neutral and your knees are pushed back. Bring your arms behind you with your thumbs pointing outward. Pull your shoulders down, and lock your lats.

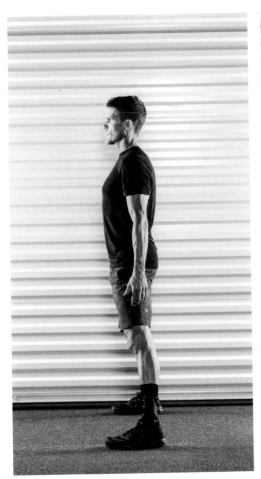 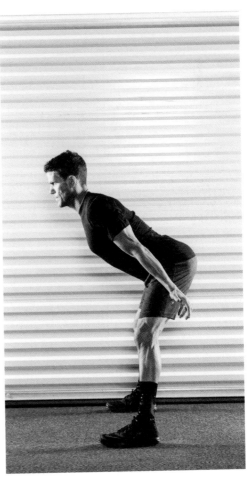

Reach out in front of you, extending your arms fully, and create a sphere of tension, and look through it while packing your shoulders down and keeping your chin pulled back. Your whole body should be engaged in the act of tensioning.

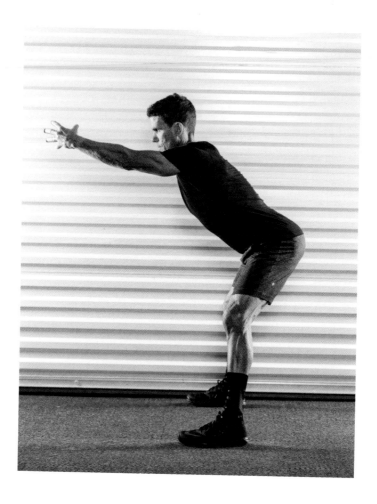

> HIP HINGE

Hinging from the hips is one of the most important movement patterns to master because it's how we lift almost everything off the ground—kids, groceries, lumber . . . you name it. It's also the most important building-block movement for the workouts later on, when you learn how to perform dead lifts and kettlebell swings, and other hinging exercises.

Proper hinging comes from the hips, not the back. If your hips and glutes aren't the driving force, then you're bending over through your back, and that's a bad pattern for lifting anything—and a good way to get injured.

Start your hip hinge by standing with your feet shoulder-width apart, with feet pointed straight ahead, begin corkscrewing your feet into the floor, squeezing your glutes and pulling your ribs down. Bend your arms at 90 degrees, pull your shoulders down, and lock your lats.

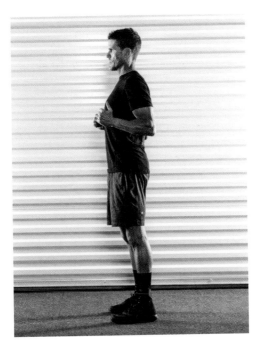

Take in a sniff of air, and brace your core. Now actively pull your hips behind you. Think of your hips going back and your chest coming forward, equal and opposite. Try to keep your shins vertical, with your knees slightly bent. From the bottom position, focus on staying braced and using your glutes to thrust your hips forward back to the starting position.

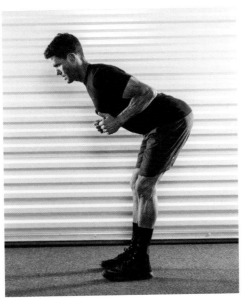

> LUNGE STRETCH (WITH KNEE DROP)

The lunge stretch with knee drops, a two-part movement, are especially important for anyone who sits a lot because sitting shortens and tightens the hip flexors and psoas muscles, which can cause lower back and hip pain. The lunge stretch is all about countering those ill effects. If you sit a lot at work, set an alarm once an hour, get up, and do a good, long lunge stretch.

Part two of the lunge stretch is the knee drops, which you'll do from the lunging position. Knee drops are an active stretch of the hip flexors, and they teach dynamic movement while holding tension.

Begin in a split stance. Keep your hips square with your front knee slightly bent. Squeeze your back glute, and scissor tension your feet, pulling your front foot backward while pushing tension forward with your back foot—scissoring them—creating a stable pelvis and better balance.

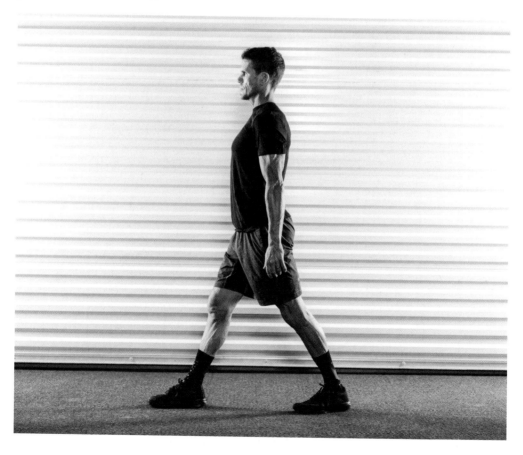

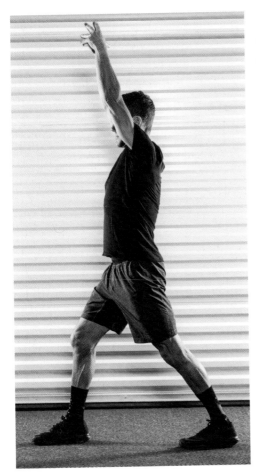

Create a sphere of tension, and continue to reach up until your arms are straight above you. Make sure as you're bringing your arms up that you're lengthening straight up and not going back into extension. Keep your eyes forward with your chin pulled back and your back straight.

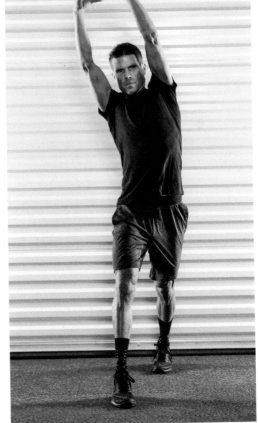

Now, take in a deep breath, and as you slowly bend to the side toward your front leg, let the air out while squeezing the back glute, keeping your arms fully extended and lengthening the opposite side of your body as much as possible. With every breath in keep reaching higher.

Bring your arms back to the center, and, keeping tension, drop your back knee to the floor (or as close as you can get) without your front knee traveling forward. Then return to the starting position.

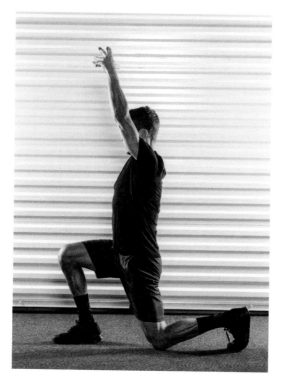

> WOODPECKER HOLDS, WOODPECKER HINGES, AND WOODPECKER ROTATIONS

When Eric Goodman introduced this movement to me, we struggled to find a descriptive name for it. Then I remembered a toy from my childhood—one of those wooden woodpeckers that hinged forward and back, dipping its beak into water over and over. That image of a perfect hinge gave birth to the name. Be mindful of your posture here, and pay close attention to how much your glutes become activated and your hamstrings lengthened.

WOODPECKER HOLDS

As with the lunge stretch, begin the woodpecker in a split stance. Extend your arms straight behind you, lock in your lats, keep your shoulders packed down, and keep your chin back. Sniff in some air, and brace your abs.

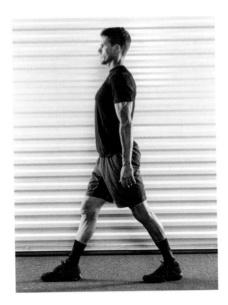

Now, slowly bring your chest forward and, at the same time, drive the left hip back. Your right leg should be slightly bent with the shin vertical, and your left leg should be straight. To put more emphasis on your front glute and hamstring, slowly raise up on the back toe as if doing a calf raise—80 percent of your weight should be on that front right foot. You should feel the glute in your front leg start to activate. Slowly reach your arms out in front of you to create a sphere of tension, and hold for at least ten seconds. (You should feel your glute start to activate.)

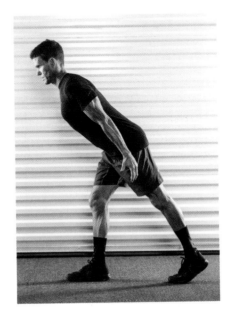

WOODPECKER HINGES

From the sphere of tension, bring your arms back to 90 degrees (as if you're rowing). Now, slowly hinge forward and back through your hips making sure the movement is coming from your hip and not your back. Keep your core braced at all times.

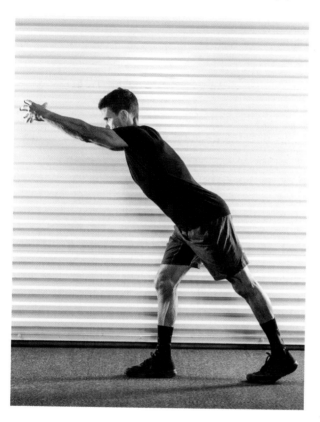

WOODPECKER ROTATIONS

While in the bottom of the hinge, reach out with both arms in front of you, creating a sphere of tension. Slowly rotate over six to eight inches to your side and over your front leg. Put all your focus on keeping tension and actively pulling your arms back to the center with your front glute. You should feel your glute activate.

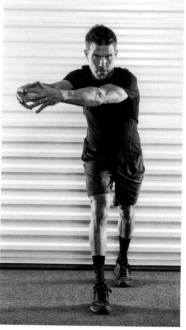

> BODY WEIGHT SQUAT

Squatting is a fundamental human movement that most of us don't do anymore. Why should we? How often do you go digging for roots like our ancestors did? Or squat down low to plant rice or potatoes, and then harvest them come the season? The problem is when you stop squatting, you lose mobility, flexibility, and strength. Too often the default pattern becomes bending over, rounding your back, and using joints and muscles not designed to take load. And over time that creates pain.

Practicing an unweighted squat will help you regain mobility in your ankles, hip flexors, adductors, and hips, and it will also strengthen your glutes and quads. It won't take long before the movement becomes natural again. Later you'll learn progressions of the body weight squat such as the goblet squat and the Bulgarian split squat.

Start with your feet shoulder-width apart or slightly wider. Looking straight ahead while keeping your chin pulled back, pull your arms back into a 90 degree position and pull your shoulders down. Now, begin corkscrewing your feet into the floor, squeezing your glutes, and pulling your ribs down. Take a sniff of air through your nose, and brace your abs.

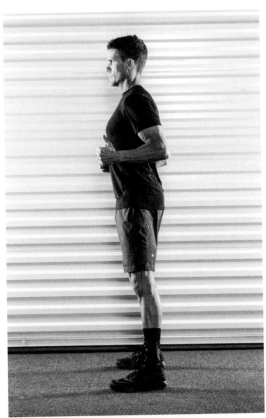

Initiate the squat by slowly pulling your hips back while pushing your arms straight out in front of you, turning your thumbs outward to help lock your shoulders and create a stiff upper back. Go down slowly to avoid air dropping; otherwise, you'll lose tension and you will default into a bad, loose pattern. Keep your shins as vertical as possible, trying to keep your weight centered over the midfoot, and drive your knees out over your toes (but not past them). Drop down as low as possible (and is safe) while maintaining stability and without letting your heels come off the ground or your back round. Be patient and consistent. Your mobility will quickly improve.

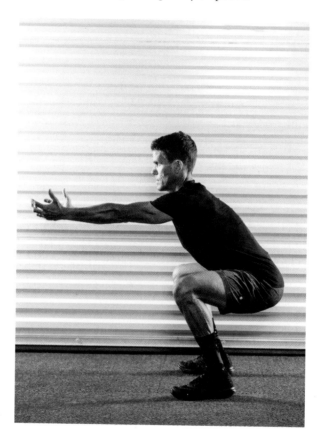

Once you've squatted as low as you are able, rise out of the bottom using a powerful hip drive to return to the starting position. Squeeze your quads and glutes and brace your core at the top of every rep. Then do a quick check of your posture before the next squat.

CORE ROUND

> JANDA CRUNCH

There are a lot of different ways to do a crunch, but my favorite is the Janda crunch. Created by Czech physiologist Vladimir Janda, this exercise isolates the abs by virtually eliminating the hip flexor's involvement.

Start by lying on your back, with your knees bent 90 degrees, feet flat on the floor. Extend your arms next to your hips, palms down flat on the floor. Take a sniff of air, squeeze your glutes, push your feet into the floor, and pull your ribs down. Now, as you come up into a crunch, let all the air out of your belly and contract your abs with maximum tension.

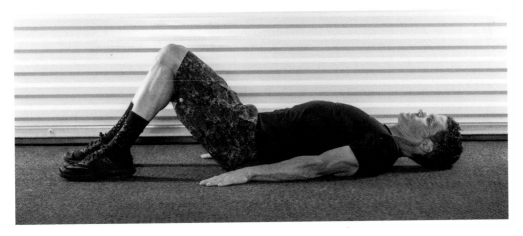

As you reach the top of the crunch, drive your hands into the floor, creating as much tension as possible. Hold five seconds at the top, then slowly return to the starting point.

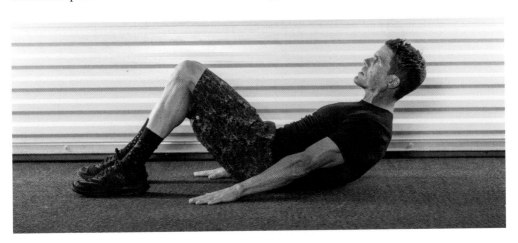

> OBLIQUE ROLL

To me, one of the best ways to work the oblique muscles in a dynamic way is this exercise. It also helps you learn how to maintain a neutral spine dynamically and creates stiffness in your core.

Start on your back, with a ball between your legs and hips at 90 degrees. Place your left arm out to the side and your right arm straight up, fully extended. Pull your ribs down, tuck your pelvis, and take in a sniff of air and brace your abs.

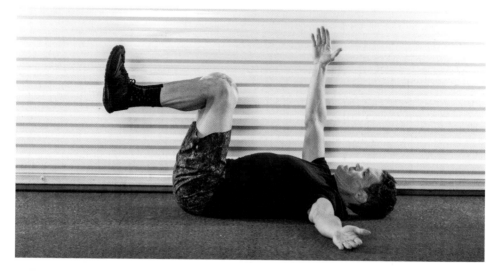

Now slowly, as one unit, roll to your left side, keeping ribs locked down and core braced. Keep your arms straight. Go down until your knees and arms are about one inch from the ground. Now, rebrace your core and, using no momentum, focus on using your obliques to come up as one unit to the starting position. Hips and shoulders should move at the exact same time, and knees and feet should stay about six inches apart.

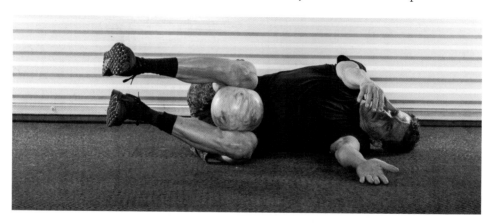

> SIDE PLANK

Side planks work lateral stability and incorporate the quadratus lumborum to greatly help stabilize the spine. As with all planks, I will have you do short ten to fifteen all-out tension holds.

Lie on your side with one arm underneath you at 90 degrees. Bring your top foot forward slightly in front of your bottom foot. Take a sniff of air, brace your abs, squeeze your glutes, pull your ribs down, keep your chin pulled back, and lock in, creating as much tension as possible from the neck down. Hold for the prescribed amount of time.

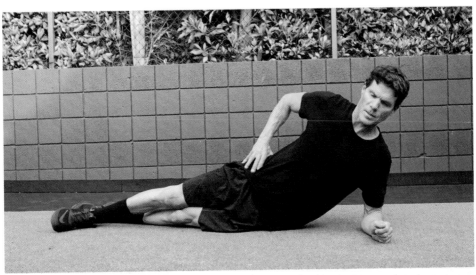

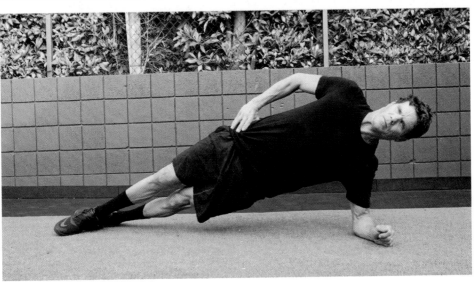

These movements and activation exercises are the building blocks of the Rebound program, so be mindful and take your time learning them and focus on perfect technique. Now it's time to begin training. Here's a rundown of your first four weeks:

- You're going to train three days per week. Never strength train two days in a row.

- In every workout during Movement Practice you'll do two circuits, a short cardio workout, and then finish with stretching, smashing, and rolling.

RECOVERY

The following are the stretches, rolls, and smashes you'll do during Recovery sessions. I've organized them in the same three groups of four that you'll do every week. Look, no way around it, it's gonna hurt some. But it's the good kind of pain, the sort that helps heal you one stretch, roll, or smash at a time.

EQUIPMENT: You'll need a bench (or your couch), a peanut ball, kettlebell, hard softball, foam roller, and, for the diaphragm smash, a volleyball or other softer ball of that size. If you don't have a peanut ball, buy two lacrosse balls, stuff them in a sock, and tie it closed.

DAY ONE

> T-SPINE SMASH—PEANUT BALL

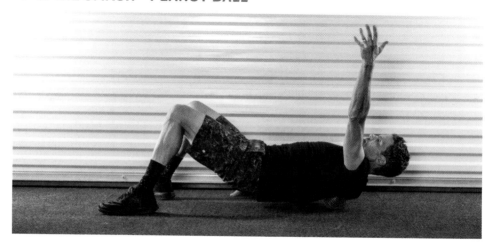

This smash is a must-do for golfers looking to increase their upper back mobility. Using a peanut ball, you'll get both sides of the spine as you smash. This smash might hurt, but you can control the pain by how much body weight you put on the ball.

Start on your back, with the peanut ball at the base of your neck. If you can, bridge up to put more weight on the ball, letting the ball sink into your tissue. Take in and then let out a deep breath of air. Now, bring your arms up and behind you, fully extended, and oscillate them. This causes the ball to smash into the tissue. Do five oscillations, then move the ball an inch or so lower, repeat, continuing down until you've made your way to midback.

> COUCH STRETCH

Stand in front of a couch (or bench) with your back to the low end of couch. Put your left foot behind you, on the couch, and take a small hop forward with your right foot. Drop your left knee gently to the floor (use a pillow or pad if needed), keeping it as close to the couch as possible. Take hold of the couch or bench behind you for balance. Square your hips, and slightly push them forward while keeping your posture as vertical as you can. Start taking in slow, deep breaths and exhaling slowly. Squeeze your back glute and make sure you keep your ribs pulled down. You should feel a stretch in the left quad. Now, create tension anywhere you can, and push your bent knee into the floor for five seconds. Exhale and release, and go a little deeper into the stretch for ten seconds, then do another contraction. Continue for two minutes, then switch legs.

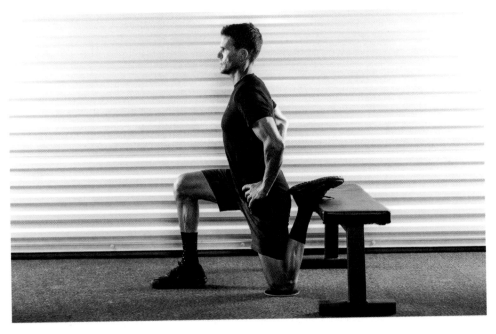

> PSOAS SMASH—KETTLEBELL

For this smash you'll use the handle of a kettlebell, which will dig deep into your psoas and iliacus, muscles that tighten in the front of your body and can cause back pain; alternatively, you could use a hard softball. Placement of the kettlebell handle is key to this smash, so pay close attention to the photo. Start with the kettlebell handle turned at a slight angle, with the top pointing inward. Slowly lower yourself on top of the handle, placing it just above your pelvic bone. Allow it to sink into your pelvic floor, taking full breaths in and out. As you do it you'll feel the kettlebell handle sink deeper into the muscles and allow them to slowly release. Once you've reached the point where you feel you have achieved more mobility, try bringing your knee up to your side or windshield wiping the foot. Then switch sides.

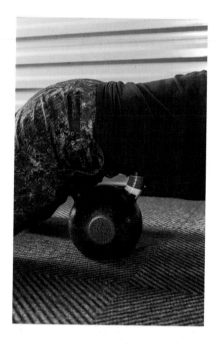

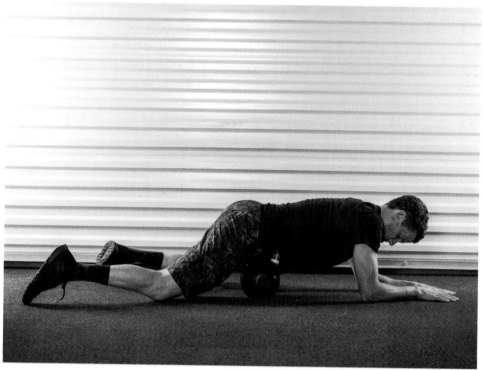

> GLUTE/TFL SMASH—HARD SOFTBALL

Sit down on the floor with the ball underneath the middle of your glute. Cross your opposing leg (opposite the glute the ball's siting on), and lean back on your elbows. Start rolling your glute over the ball back and forth, keeping as much of your body weight on it as you can tolerate. Be mindful of your breathing, with slow, long exhales, allowing yourself to sink deeper into the ball. After about two minutes roll the ball on the outside of your hip (the TFL). Use your arms to balance you, circling around the muscles that insert on the lateral hip bone. Do this for two minutes, then switch to the other glute-hip.

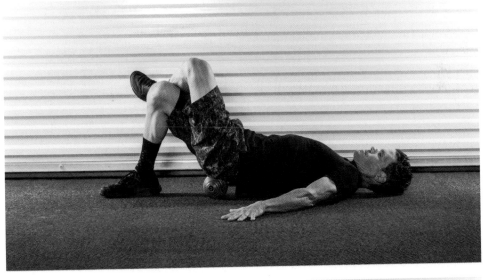

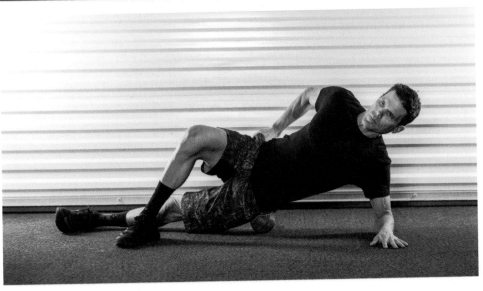

DAY TWO

> PEC SMASH—HARD SOFTBALL

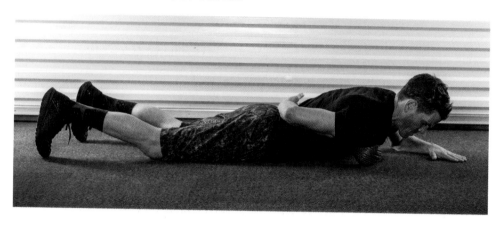

Lie on your stomach, and insert the ball into the space between where your right pec and right shoulder meet. Now, if you can, put your right arm, bent, behind you. This helps put more weight and pressure on the pec.

Take in a deep breath, then let it out. Now, smash the pec from the collarbone to the lower pec by going back and forth and in circles over the ball. Make sure you breathe throughout. After 2 minutes switch sides.

> HAMSTRING SMASH— HARD SOFTBALL

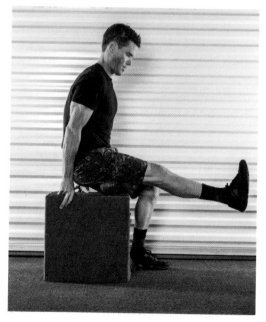

Sit on a box or a coffee table—something hard and stable with no cushion or give. Place the ball right below your sit bone where your hamstring and butt meet. Put as much weight or pressure as you feel comfortable, fully extending the knee out and in while also going back and forth, working your way down toward the knee as you go. Once you reach the knee, start moving the ball side to side up the leg toward your sit bone. After 2 minutes switch sides.

> DIAPHRAGM SMASH—SIX-INCH BALL

The diaphragm smash loosens abdominal muscles, which can help relieve back pain and improve breathing.

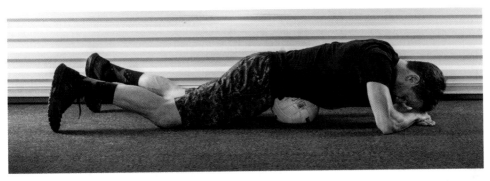

Lie down on top of the ball centered in your stomach, an inch or two below the belly button. Your arms should be in front of you. Take a full breath in and a full breath out, and slowly begin to trace the ball around the whole outer rib cage and down to the pelvis. After a minute change directions for one more minute.

> HAMSTRING STRETCH

Tight hamstrings deter proper hinging and can force you to round your back, which can cause lower back pain.

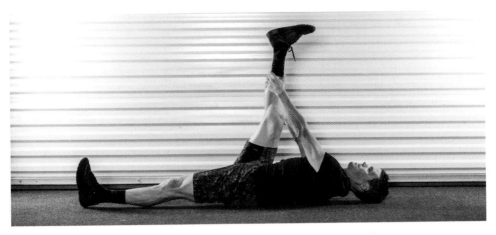

Lie on your back, with one leg extended up and your knee locked or slightly bent. Grab your leg at the calf. Pull your leg toward your head until you're getting a good stretch. Now, take in some air, and push your leg against your hands and your hands against your leg, contracting the hamstring muscle for five seconds. Exhale and release the contraction and pull the hamstring deeper into the stretch. Hold for ten seconds. Repeat for two minutes, then switch legs.

DAY THREE

> LAT-TO-ROTATOR CUFF ROLL—FOAM ROLLER

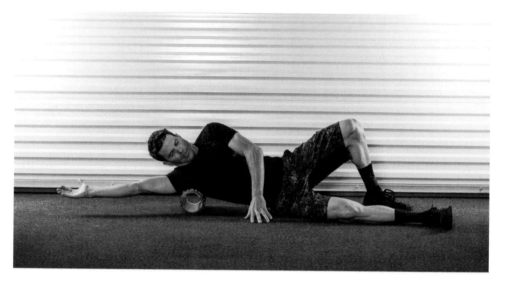

This roll will help you get back shoulder mobility. Rolling your lats might be painful at first, but you can control the pain level by how much body weight you put on the roller.

Lay on your side with a foam roller right above your hip. Angle your body so you start with the back side of the body, your arm extended as much above your head as your mobility allows. Start by taking in a deep breath and letting it out, then work your way rolling up to your armpit, then back down toward your stomach. If you find a spot that feels especially nasty, crunchy, or tight, roll on it as long as it takes to get a release. Go two minutes on each side.

> PIGEON STRETCH

For a lot of people, especially athletes who may be tight from so much exercise, just getting into the pigeon stretch can be a real challenge. I suggest starting out using a bench or a table to support you, as in the photo. But if your hip flexors are already pretty flexible, by all means do your pigeon stretches on the floor.

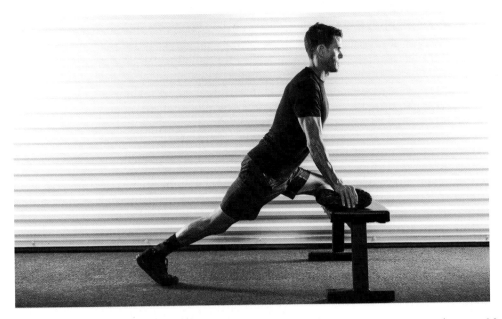

Lay your left shin (foot to your knee) on a bench or couch, bent at or close to 90 degrees. Extend your right leg back behind you. Keep your back flat, with your chin neutral. Take in a long breath of air, let it out, and lean forward as far as you can without breaking form. You should feel a stretch in your left glute and hip. Do ten short forward pulses here, using breathing to pace and control the stretch.

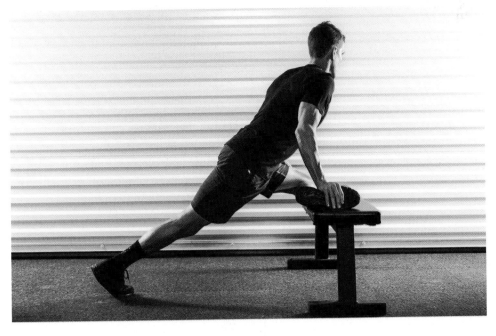

Next, rotate your body to the left, extending your right hand out past your left knee, again, maintaining your good form. Do ten forward pulses here.

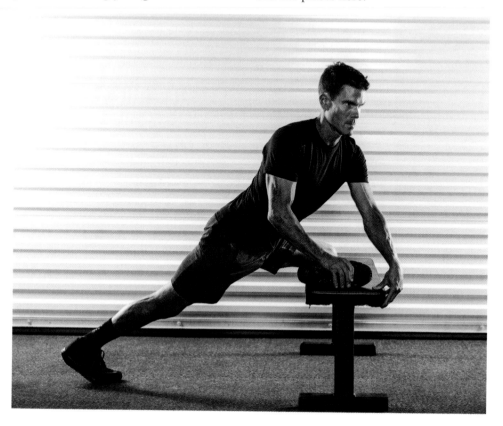

Next, rotate your body to the right, extending your left hand past your left foot. Do ten forward pulses.

> ADDUCTOR STRETCH

The adductors are the muscles on the inside of your thighs that are often underused and tight and become big problem areas for many people, from desk jockeys to professional athletes.

Place your left heel on a platform, your body facing forward, your toes pointed upward. Lean in sideways toward your foot that's on the platform. You should feel a stretch in your inner thigh/groin. While doing this stretch try moving your foot in different directions to stretch different parts of your adductors. After five seconds release and go deeper into the stretch.

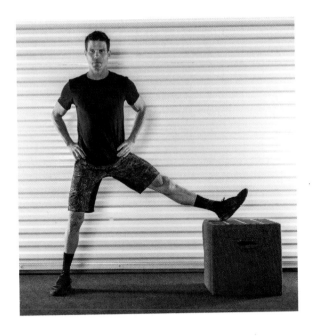

> CALF ROLL—FOAM ROLLER

A terrific foam-rolling exercise for those of us who have restricted ankle joint mobility and tightness in the calves and Achilles. By rolling, you're freeing the restricted tissue by smashing with the foam roller all the way from the Achilles to the top of the calf behind the knee.

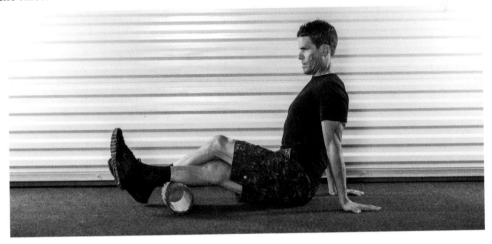

Start on the floor, sitting up, with your Achilles against the foam roller. Place your free leg on top of your shin to add pressure.

Slowly roll up the mid-calf finding tight spots. Roll for two minutes per leg.

Circuit One—2x

Ankle Mobility	Bird Dogs	T-spine Rotations	Eight-Point Plank	Founder	Hip Hinge
10 pulses outward, middle and inward for each ankle ➤	7x alternating sides ➤	7x per side ➤	2x 10-second holds, 10-second rest between sets ➤	2x 10-second holds (maximum full-body tension), 10-second rest between sets ➤	10x

Circuit Two—2x

Lunge Stretch	Woodpecker	Body Weight Squat	Wide Founder
2x 15-second holds, per side ➤	2x 15-second holds, per side ➤	10x ➤	2x 10-second holds (maximum full-body tension), 10-second rest between sets

Cardio

20 minutes of low-intensity, base-building cycling, jogging on the treadmill, elliptical—any machine that gets your heart rate up to your MAHR or 60–70% exertion.

Recovery

Couch Stretch	T-Spine Smash
2 minutes per leg ➤	4 minutes

Circuit One—2x

Ankle Mobility	Bird Dogs	T-Spine Rotations	Eight-Point Plank	Founder	Hip Hinge
10 pulses outward, middle and inward for each ankle ➤	7x alternating sides ➤	7x per side ➤	2x 10-second holds, 10-second rest between sets ➤	2x 10-second holds (maximum full-body tension), 10-second rest between sets ➤	10x

Circuit Two—2x

Lunge Stretch	Woodpecker	Body Weight Squat	Wide Founder
2x 15-second holds, per side ➤	2x 15-second holds, per side ➤	10x ➤	2x 10-second holds (maximum full-body tension), 10-second rest between sets

Cardio

20 minutes of low-intensity, base-building cycling, jogging on the treadmill, elliptical—any machine that gets your heart rate up to your MAHR or 60–70% exertion.

Recovery

Glute/TFL Smash	Psoas Smash
2 minutes per side ➤	2 minutes per side

Circuit One—2x

Ankle Mobility	Bird Dogs	T-Spine Rotations	Eight-Point Plank	Founder	Hip Hinge
10 pulses outward, middle and inward for each ankle ➤	7x alternating sides ➤	7x per side ➤	2x 10-second holds, 10-second rest between sets ➤	2x 10-second holds (maximum full-body tension), 10-second rest between sets ➤	10x

Circuit Two—2x

Lunge Stretch	Woodpecker	Body Weight Squat	Wide Founder
2x 15-second holds, per side ➤	2x 15-second holds, per side ➤	10x ➤	2x 10-second holds (maximum full-body tension), 10-second rest between sets

Cardio

20 minutes of low-intensity, base-building cycling, jogging on the treadmill, elliptical—any machine that gets your heart rate up to your MAHR or 60–70% exertion. **Optional:** choose two machines and go 10 minutes on each.

Recovery

Pec Smash	Hamstring Smash
2 minutes per side, find sticky spots between the pec and shoulder ➤	2 minutes per side, remember to contract for 5 seconds then go deeper into the stretch.

Circuit One—2x

Ankle Mobility	Bird Dogs	T-Spine Rotations	Eight-Point Plank	Founder	Hip Hinge
10 pulses outward, middle and inward for each ankle ➤	10x alternating sides ➤	10x per side ➤	3x 10-second holds, 10-second rest between sets ➤	3x 10-second holds, 10-second rest between sets ➤	12x

Circuit Two—2x

Lunge Stretch	Woodpecker	Body Weight Squat	Wide Founder
3x 10-second holds, per side ➤	3x 10-second holds, per side ➤	12x ➤	3x 10-second holds (maximum full-body tension), 10-second rest between sets

Cardio

25 minutes of low-intensity, base-building cycling, jogging on the treadmill, elliptical—any machine that gets your heart rate up to your MAHR or 60–70% exertion.

Recovery

Hamstring Stretch	Diaphragm Smash
2 minutes per leg ➤	4 minutes

Circuit One—2x

Ankle Mobility	Bird Dogs	T-Spine Rotations	Eight-Point Plank	Founder	Hip Hinge
10 pulses outward, middle and inward for each ankle ➤	10x alternating sides ➤	10x per side ➤	3x 10-second holds, 10-second rest between sets ➤	3x 10-second holds, 10-second rest between sets ➤	12x

Circuit Two—2x

Lunge Stretch	Woodpecker	Body Weight Squat	Wide Founder
3x 10-second holds, per side ➤	3x 10-second holds, per side, 10 second rest between sets ➤	12x ➤	3x 10-second holds (full-body tension), 10-second rest between sets

Cardio

25 minutes of low-intensity, base-building cycling, jogging on the treadmill, elliptical—
any machine that gets your heart rate up to your MAHR or 60–70% exertion

Recovery

Lat-to-Rotator Smash	Pigeon Stretch
2 minutes per side ➤	2 minutes per side

Circuit One—2x

Ankle Mobility	Bird Dogs	T-Spine Rotations	Eight-Point Plank	Founder	Hip Hinge
10 pulses outward, middle and inward for each ankle ➤	10x alternating sides ➤	10x per side ➤	3x 10-second holds, 10-second rest between sets ➤	3x 10-second holds, 10-second rest between sets ➤	12x

Circuit Two—2x

Lunge Stretch	Woodpecker	Body Weight Squat	Wide Founder
3x 10-second holds, per side ➤	3x 10-second holds, per side, 10-second rest inbetween sets ➤	12x ➤	3x 10-second holds (maximum full-body tension), 10-second rest between sets

Cardio

25 minutes of low-intensity, base-building cycling, jogging on the treadmill, elliptical—any machine that gets your heart rate up to your MAHR or 60–70% exertion.

Recovery

Adductor Stretch	Calf Smash
2 minutes per side ➤	2 minutes per side

Circuit One—2x

Ankle Mobility	Bird Dogs	T-Spine Rotations	Eight-Point Plank	Founder	Hip Hinge
10 pulses outward, middle and inward for each ankle ➤	10x alternating sides ➤	10x per side ➤	2x 15-second holds with knees off the ground, 10 second rest between sets ➤	2x 15-second holds, 10-second rest between sets ➤	12x

Circuit Two—2x

Lunge Stretch + Knee Drops	Woodpecker	Body Weight Squat	Wide Founder
15-second holds, then 7x knee drops, per side ➤	• 10-second holds • 10x hinges • 10-second holds, per side ➤	12x ➤	2x 15-second holds (maximum full-body tension), 10-second rest between sets

Cardio

25 minutes of low-intensity, base-building cycling, jogging on the treadmill, elliptical—any machine that gets your heart rate up to your MAHR or 60–70% exertion.

Recovery

Couch Stretch	T-Spine Smash
2 minutes per leg ➤	4 minutes

Circuit One—2x

Ankle Mobility	Bird Dogs	T-Spine Rotations	Eight-Point Plank	Founder	Hip Hinge
10 pulses outward, middle and inward for each ankle ➤	10x alternating sides ➤	10x per side ➤	2x 15-second holds with knees off the ground, 10-second rest between sets ➤	2x 15-second holds, 10-second rest between sets ➤	12x

Circuit Two—2x

Lunge Stretch + Knee Drops	Woodpecker	Body Weight Squat	Wide Founder
15-second holds, then 7x knee drops, per side ➤	• 1x 10-second holds • 10x hinges • 1x 10-second hold, per side ➤	12x ➤	2x 15-second holds, 10-second rest between sets

Cardio

25 minutes of low-intensity, base-building cycling, jogging on the treadmill, elliptical— any machine that gets your heart rate up to your MAHR or 60–70% exertion.

Recovery

Glute/TFL Smash	Psoas Smash
2 minutes per side ➤	2 minutes per side

Circuit One—2x

Ankle Mobility	Bird Dogs	T-Spine Rotations	Eight-Point Plank	Founder	Hip Hinge
10 pulses outward, middle and inward for each ankle ➤	10x alternating sides ➤	10x per side ➤	2x 15-second holds with knees off the ground, 10-second rest between sets ➤	2x 15-second holds, 10-second rest between sets ➤	12x

Circuit Two—2x

Lunge Stretch + Knee Drops	Woodpecker	Body Weight Squat	Wide Founder
15-second holds, then 7x knee drops, per side ➤	• 10-second holds • 10x hinges • 10-second holds, per side ➤	12x ➤	2x 15-second holds (maximum full-body tension), 10-second rest between sets

Cardio

25 minutes of low-intensity, base-building cycling, jogging on the treadmill, elliptical—any machine that gets your heart rate up to your MAHR or 60–70% exertion.

Recovery

Pec Smash	Hamstring Smash
2 minutes per side ➤	2 minutes per side

Circuit One—2x

Ankle Mobility	Bird Dogs	T-Spine Rotations	Eight-Point Plank	Founder	Hip Hinge
10 pulses outward, middle and inward for each ankle ➤	10x alternating sides ➤	10x per side ➤	3x 15-second holds with knees off the ground, 10-second rest between sets ➤	3x 15-second holds, 10-second rest between sets ➤	12x

Circuit Two—2x

Lunge Stretch + Knee Drops	Woodpecker	Body Weight Squat	Wide Founder
15-second holds, then 7x knee drops, per side ➤	• 15-second holds • 10 hinges • 10 rotations, per side ➤	12x ➤	3x 15-second holds, 10-second rest between sets

Cardio

30 minutes of low-intensity, base-building cardio exercise at 60–70% exertion.

Recovery

Diaphragm Smash	Hamstring Smash
4 minutes, roll slowly and be mindful of your breathing ➤	2 minutes per leg, 10-second stretch, 5-second contraction, go deeper into the stretch

Circuit One—2x

Ankle Mobility	Bird Dogs	T-Spine Rotations	Eight-Point Plank	Founder	Hip Hinge
10 pulses outward, middle and inward for each ankle ➤	10x alternating sides ➤	10x per side ➤	3x 15-second holds with knees off the ground, 10-second rest between sets ➤	3x 15-second holds, 10-second rest between sets ➤	12x (go slow, chest forward)

Circuit Two—2x

Lunge Stretch + Knee Drops	Woodpecker	Body Weight Squat	Wide Founder
10-second holds, then 7x knee drops, per side ➤	• 15-second holds • 10 hinges • 10 rotations, per side ➤	12x ➤	3x 15-second holds, 10-second rest between sets

Cardio

30 minutes of low-intensity, base-building cardio at 60–70% exertion.
Optional: Use two different cardio machines and go 15 minutes on each.

Recovery

Pigeon Stretch	Lat-to-Rotator Cuff Roll
2 minutes per side ➤	2 minutes per side, roll slowly over sticky spots

Circuit One—2x

Ankle Mobility	Bird Dogs	T-Spine Rotations	Eight-Point Plank	Founder	Hip Hinge
10 pulses outward, middle and inward for each ankle ➤	10x alternating sides ➤	10x per side ➤	2x 15-second holds with knees off the ground, 10-second rest between sets ➤	2x 15-second holds, 10-second rest between ➤	12x

Circuit Two—2x

Lunge Stretch + Knee Drops	Woodpecker	Body Weight Squat	Wide Founder
15-second holds, then 7x knee drops, per side ➤	• 1x 10-second holds • 10 hinges • 1x 10-second holds, per side ➤	12x ➤	3x 15-second holds, (focus on creating full-body tensioning), 10-second rest between sets

Cardio

30 minutes of low-intensity, base-building cardio at 60–70% exertion.
Optional: Choose three machines and go 5 minutes on each, 2x.

Recovery

Adductor Stretch	Calf Smash
2 minutes per side ➤	2 minutes per side, rolling slowly over tight spots

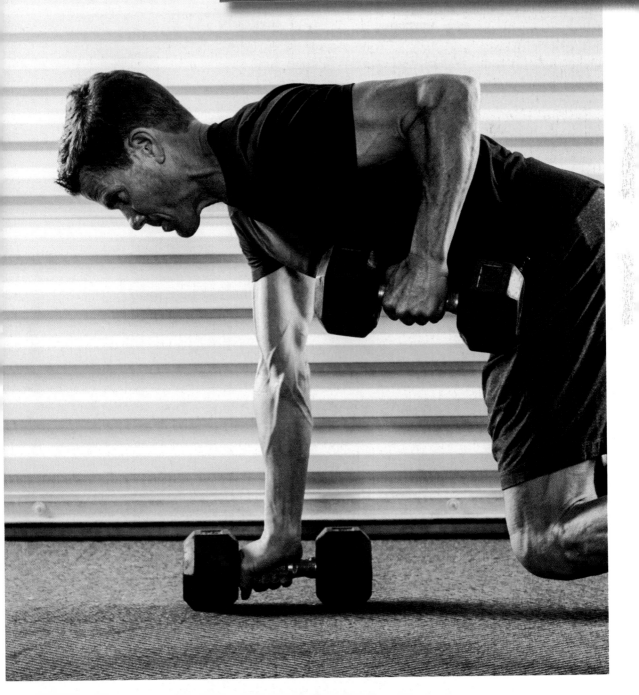

PART THREE
THE WORKOUTS

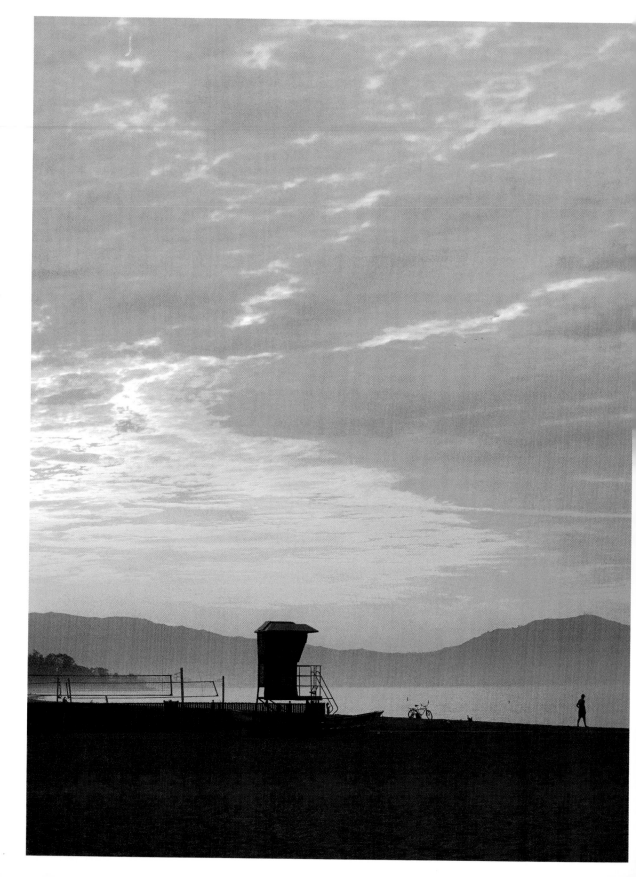

CHAPTER EIGHT: EAST BEACH

SOMETIMES YOU JUST GET LUCKY IN LIFE. You're at the right place at the right time. And for me the right place was East Beach in Santa Barbara and the right time was 1977. I was twelve back then and had a neighbor who was, at that time, the best high school volleyball player anywhere. He'd go on to become an Olympic gold medalist. His name is Karch Kiraly. Karch is a few years older than me, but most summer mornings and on weekends we went up to East Beach, a volleyball Mecca, where the best players went to play.

Karch's strong work ethic was a big influence on me. We'd play from early in the morning till dusk, and at the end of every day Karch, professional players like John Hanley and John Stevenson, and I would race through the deep sand from East Beach to Stearns Wharf and back. The loser had to do it again. That's when I learned how much I hated to lose. So East Beach is where I built my foundation as an athlete, and so you too, dear reader, will begin rebuilding yours with the East Beach workout.

Before we begin I want to check in with you and make sure you're moving well enough now to begin lifting weights. Have the four weeks of retraining your movement patterns got you hinging and squatting properly? Are you getting your core stiff and activated? Or you're still not quite getting it? You still have pain in a knee or shoulder, your lower back hurts, and cardio-wise you're struggling to make it for the full twenty-five minutes of low-intensity exercise? Listen to your body. If you don't feel ready to lift weights, keep going with movement practice a little while longer.

And how's the eating going? Is cutting down on sugar tough? Keep at it—it's important. If cutting down on carbs was the harder part, relief is in sight. You're going to start doing some higher-intensity interval training in this chapter, so you get to add a few more grams of carbs back into your diet.

Try to eat them just before or right after your workout. (Or, if you're training longer, perhaps during workout.) For instance, if I'm going to train at three in the afternoon, an hour before I'd have a small snack such as one-half of a banana with almond butter. Then for my postworkout I would drink or eat 10 to 20 grams of protein and around 30 grams of carbs to refuel. I always prefer real food—sweet potato with my spinach and grilled salmon, whole-grain toast with my broccolini and eggs—but for the sake of convenience, there are good recovery drinks on the market, and they certainly do the trick. I recommend recovery drinks that have a three-to-one ratio of carbs to protein.

A quick note about your training schedule. Every month you start a new workout that lasts four weeks. Your first training day of a new week (be it Monday, Tuesday, or whatever day you train) I've named "Day One." Your second training day is "Day Two," and the third day, you guessed it, "Day Three." Day One and Day Three workouts are nearly identical, whereas Day Two goes back to working on your movement patterns.

How much weight should you use while training? Here are a few general guidelines:

- When you're first learning an exercise, choose weights that seem light. If you can do an exercise, say ten times, and it's really easy, then, go up a little in weight. Conversely, if you can't finish the directed number of reps or you're defaulting on your form, go lighter. Don't let your ego get you injured. You need to learn how to do the exercises correctly. There's plenty of time to progress toward heavier weights.

- In Week One of each workout you'll learn some new exercises, so go lighter that week. In Week Two you won't increase the reps, but if you have your form down and feel comfortable, add a little more weight. In Week Three you'll do even fewer reps, add more weight, and you'll start getting stronger.

- Remember, do not train to failure.

Before every workout you'll begin with your Activation exercises, a warm-up that gets your body ready for strength training. There are five or six activation movements, all designed to "wake up" your body, get your core stiff, and get it ready to lift weights. You already learned most of the activation exercises in the last chapter. Note: a lot of my clients like to warm up for five to ten minutes on a cardio machine before training. You don't have to, but if you have the time, go for it. All right, you ready? Good luck at East Beach!

NEW EXERCISES

> PUSHUPS

I know. You've probably done a million pushups in your lifetime, but have you done them while corkscrewing your hands into the floor and squeezing your heels and glutes together and while keeping your pelvis tucked? If not, you're about to see how pushups can be transformed from just a pec and back exercise to a movement that teaches the whole body how to work together and build strength throughout most of the upper body.

Begin up in a perfect plank position with your hands shoulder-width apart, elbows in. Start creating tension by squeezing your heels and glutes together and corkscrewing your hands into the floor, making sure your lats are locked and your shoulders are packed down. Now take a sniff of air through your nose, and brace your abs.

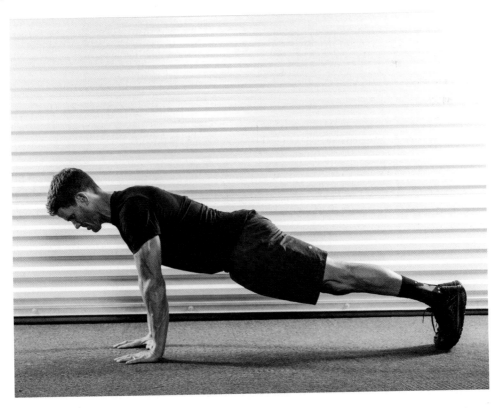

Now, while maintaining a neutral head position, actively pull yourself (don't drop down) toward the floor, keeping overall body tension. Elbows stay tucked in at your sides. Pause momentarily at the bottom, then come back up to the starting position. Check your form, rebrace, and repeat.

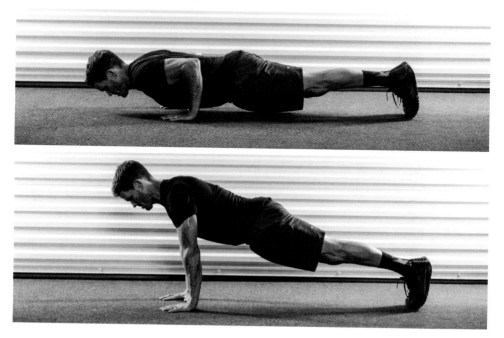

> PUSHUPS ON KNEES

Some people struggle with pushups on the floor. They're tough! If that's you, no worries, I have some choices for you. The first is doing pushups on your knees. Just follow the pushup cues above, but make sure when you're on your knees to squeeze your knees and heels together to create the needed tension. If that's still too difficult, try doing pushups on a bench. Same cues, same results.

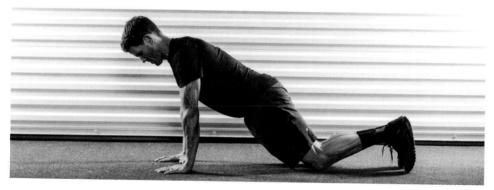

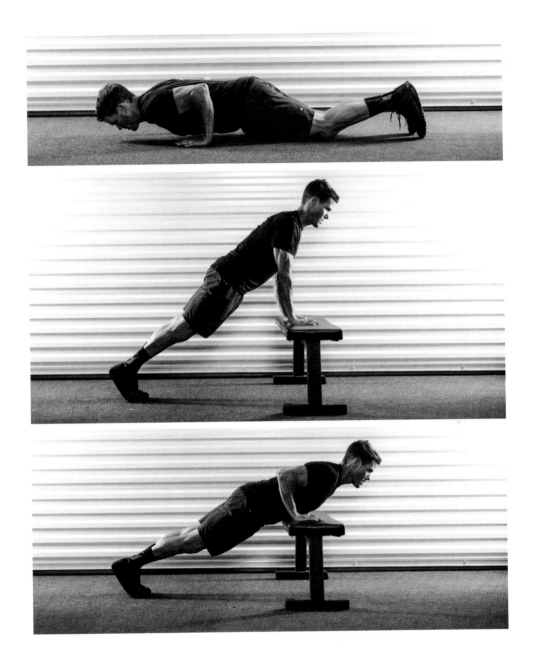

> GOBLET SQUATS

In the Movement Practice chapter you learned how to do a body weight squat. The next squat progression is to add a light weight to the movement (I prefer a kettlebell, but a dumbbell works just fine). By adding tension and holding the weight at the front of your body, a goblet squat activates your core to support the weight, and the weight will act like an anchor and help you sink into a deeper squat. That stretches the adductors, mobilizes the hips, and extends your mobility.

Tensioning is crucial before and during a goblet squat to maintain proper form. Just remember to stay braced throughout the movement, keeping your back flat, chin pulled back, your weight on the midfoot, heels touching the ground, and your shins staying as vertical as possible.

Start with your feet slightly more than shoulder-width apart, your toes pointed straight ahead or slightly out to the sides, holding the weight in both hands. Begin corkscrewing your feet, squeezing your glutes, packing your shoulders down and locking your lats. If you're using a kettlebell, "break the horns" (the handle) of the bell to create tension. Take in a sniff of air, and brace your abs.

Actively pull yourself into the squat, driving your knees outward and dropping your hips as if you're about to sit on a curb behind you. If you have sufficient mobility, you can briefly "pry" your knees apart with your elbows at the bottom of your squat. (If at any time during the squat you feel your form defaulting—your back rounds or your heels come off the ground—try to stay tight while returning to the starting position.)

Staying tight, use an explosive—but controlled—drive of the hips to power yourself back up to the starting position. Take in another sniff of air, brace again, and you're ready for your second rep.

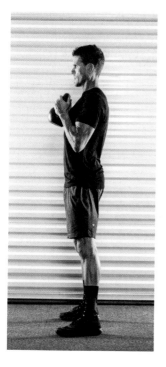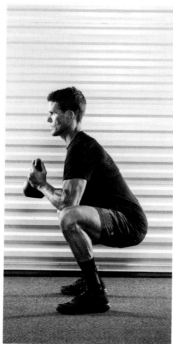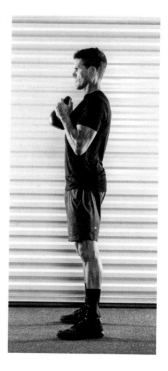

> ROMANIAN DEAD LIFT

Romanian dead lifts are hip hinges with added weight. RDLs work your hamstrings, glutes, and reinforce the whole posterior chain, and they hammer home that all-important hinge pattern. (Note: doing RDLs today might mean waking up with sore hamstrings tomorrow. Don't be alarmed—that just means you did your job.)

You'll need two kettlebells or dumbbells. Hold one in each hand. Start with your feet shoulder-width apart, feet pointed straight ahead or slightly out, and begin corkscrewing your feet into the floor. Squeeze your glutes. Pull your shoulders down, and lock your lats. Take in a sniff of air, brace your core, and, while keeping your chin pulled back, drive your hips back and chest forward, actively thinking about pushing the middle of your hamstrings behind you. As you descend, your knees should be slightly bent, weight on your midfoot. Go down until you feel a stretch in the hamstrings and glutes. The entire movement should originate from the hip, not the lower or midback.

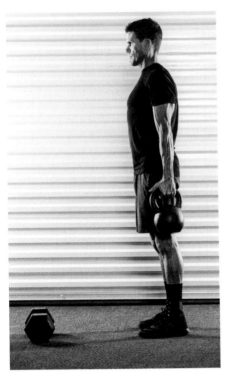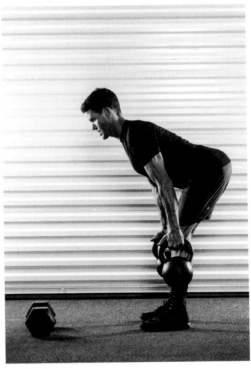

At the bottom of your lift, squeeze your glutes tighter, and use a solid hip drive to return to the start position. It's important to squeeze your quads and glutes and to rebrace your core at the top position to prevent hyperextension and spinal stress. A good cue is to think of doing a standing plank at the top of every repetition.

> BENCH ROWS

Bench rows work your lats and back and also help develop good posture and stability.

Stand next to a bench. Put one knee on the bench, bent at 90 degrees, while keeping the other foot firmly on the ground, slightly out from the bench. Put one hand on the bench, directly underneath your shoulder. Keeping your back flat, corkscrew your hand into the bench, lock in your lat, and pack in your shoulder. Take a sniff of air, and brace your abs.

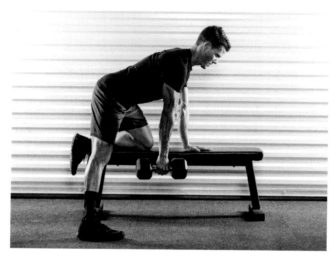

Now row or pull the weight up until your arm is bent at 90 degrees. Make sure the rest of your body remains stable, your back flat, and nothing but your arm moves. Keep your movement strict and isolated. Sniff in, and brace again at the bottom before the next rep.

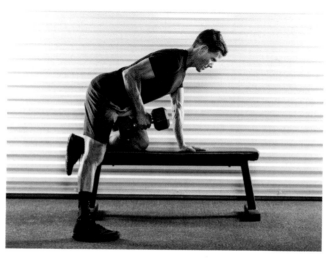

> FARMER CARRIES

Old MacDonald had a farm, and that man was strong as hell. So were his wife and his kids. Because besides plowing his fields (keeping his back flat, shoulders packed), squatting down to plant seeds, and hinging perfectly to harvest his yield, Old MacDonald and his family had to carry their pails of milk and cream a hundred yards from the barn

to the house, building grip strength, strong legs and arms, good posture, and a strong heart. That Old MacDonald was one fit dude!

Farmer carries really are as simple as just carrying either one or two dumbells at your sides, but good posture is crucial here. Use a challenging weight but one that allows you to maintain perfect form. Hinge or squat to lift the dumbbells at the middle of the handle. Make sure your shoulders stay packed down. For all carries walk about thirty seconds, but as you get stronger, start carrying heavier weight.

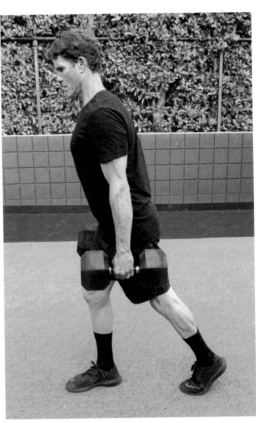

Looking straight ahead, keeping your chin back, your shoulders packed, and the weights level, walk in one direction for the designated amount of time (typically 30 seconds), turn around, then walk back, always focusing on perfect posture. Hinge or squat to put the weights down.

> THE TURKISH GETUP

If aliens came to Earth, took me back to their home planet, and asked me to show them the single-most useful exercise for the human body, they'd watch me do Turkish getups.

A lot of people are intimidated by getups because they seem so complicated—there's so many steps to them. But the very reason getups are the most useful exercise for the human body is that they are so natural. In fact, every time you get up off the floor you're pretty much doing a getup (well, minus holding a kettlebell above your head, but you'll get used to that).

You're going to learn getups in phases over the next three weeks, and as with all my clients, instead of starting with a kettlebell, I recommend you use a book or a shoe balanced on your fist, which forces you to move slowly and maintain perfect form and balance. Otherwise, the book or shoe will fall. The first week you'll learn phase one of the getup, which I call punch-up to elbow. If after a few weeks of trying you find full getups just too challenging that's okay, but stick with phase one, punch-up to elbow. It's a terrific exercise by itself.

> TURKISH GETUP: PUNCH-UP TO ELBOW (WEEK ONE)

Starting on your back, extend your right arm straight up, with the weight balanced on your fist. Position your weighted hand like you're holding a hammer (turned sideways with your thumb on top), and keep your wrist locked straight.

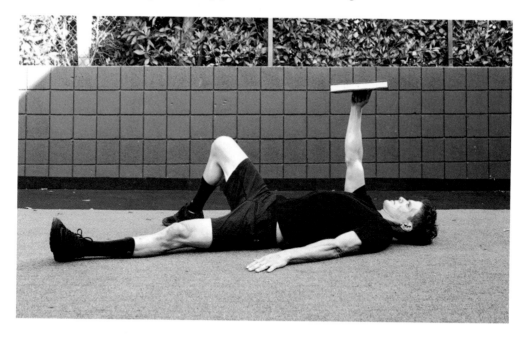

Position your left leg, as in the picture, at a 45 degree angle with your left arm on your side parallel to it. Now position your right leg slightly out to the side and bent at a 90 degree angle. You're now in the starting position.

Punch-up to the elbow focuses on using your opposite oblique—the ab muscles on your side—to pull you up. Start by taking a sniff of air through your nose, squeeze your glutes, and brace your abs. Push off your right foot and left elbow, and pivot onto the left elbow. When punching up, lead with your chest, not your head.

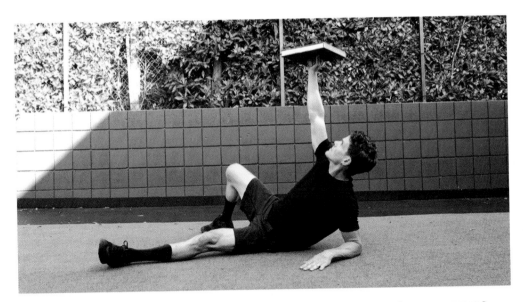

> TURKISH GETUP: PUNCH-UP TO LUNGE POSITION (WEEK TWO)

In this second week of learning the getup you're working hip mobility, shoulder stability, and more core strength as you move from the floor into a kneeling lunge position, the weight moving straight up above you. Remember to keep your eyes on the weight at all times.

Start by doing the getup from the beginning position through punch-up to elbow.

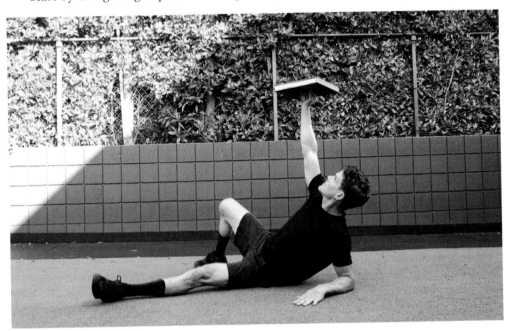

Pivot your left hand counter-clockwise (on the right side it will be clockwise) to around 90 degrees to stabilize your shoulder. Push your left hand into the ground, and push up until your left arm is locked out, never looking away from the weight. Now slowly reverse the sequence back down, carefully dropping your left elbow back to the floor to the starting position. Rebrace for the next rep.

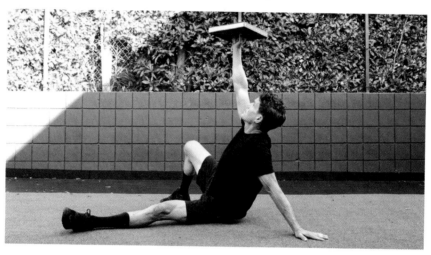

Now from there sweep your left leg underneath you like you're sitting cross-legged. Push in with your left hand and right foot, and windshield-wipe or pivot your left leg back, putting you in a kneeling position. You should be up on the tip of your toe, ready to push up into a standing position. Now look straight ahead.

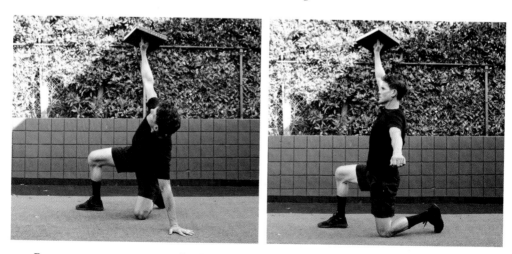

Reverse your movements back to fetal position. Sniff in, and brace again for the next rep.

> *TURKISH GETUP: KNEELING LUNGE TO STEPPING UP (WEEK THREE)*

In the third and final step of the getup the cues take you from a kneeling position with the weight held above you to standing upright, with your arm fully extended. During this third phase you're working your glutes, strengthening your legs, and creating whole-body balance and stability. Be sure to keep your eyes forward.

Start by executing a getup from the fetal position to the kneeling lunge. Make sure your back toes are pointed into the floor so you can push off with them.

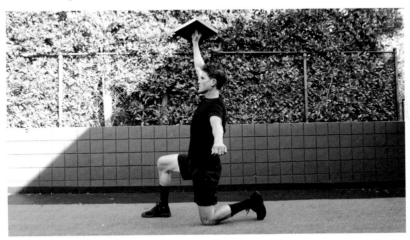

Now, take a breath, and, making sure to keep equal tension on your back toes and front heel, brace yourself and stand up, looking straight ahead as if at the horizon line.

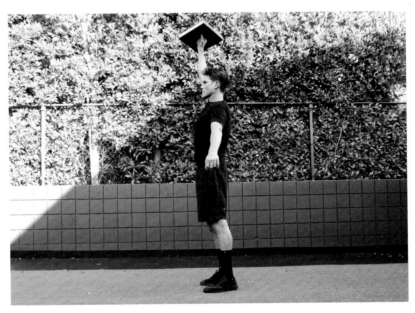

Now you're going to reverse the getup. Start by taking a big step backward with your left leg, and carefully lower your knee straight to the floor, back into lunge position.

Windshield-wiper your left foot over, and hinge your right hip out to the side as you bring your left hand down to the floor. Then bring your left leg under you, with your hand turned counter-clockwise at 90 degrees. Slide your left leg out to 45 degrees again, drop your elbow to the floor, and slowly drop back to the floor in starting position. Rebrace for the next rep.

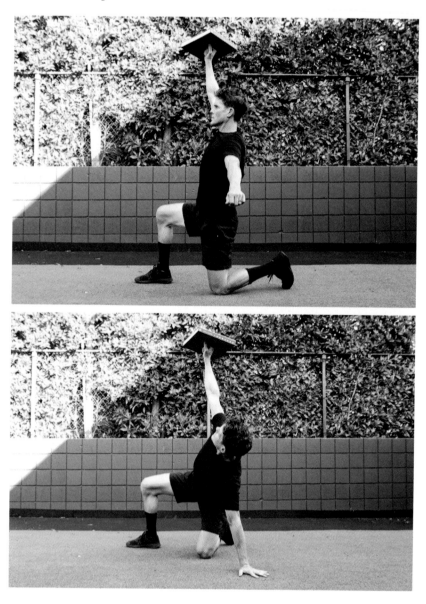

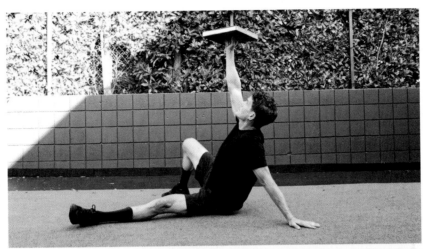

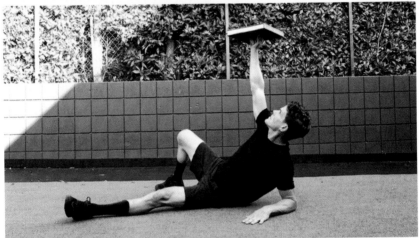

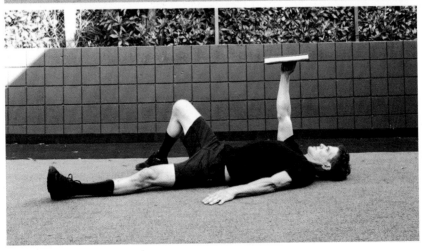

> WIDE FOUNDER WITH TRACING

When you hold a perfect wide founder, creating all that powerful tension in your glutes and abs, then trace your hands up from your hips to a full extension in front of you, you're helping your shoulders become more mobile and putting more tension in the glutes and abs. It's a great progression from the wide founder.

Start in a wide founder with your arms behind you. Corkscrew your feet into the ground, sniff in, and brace your core.

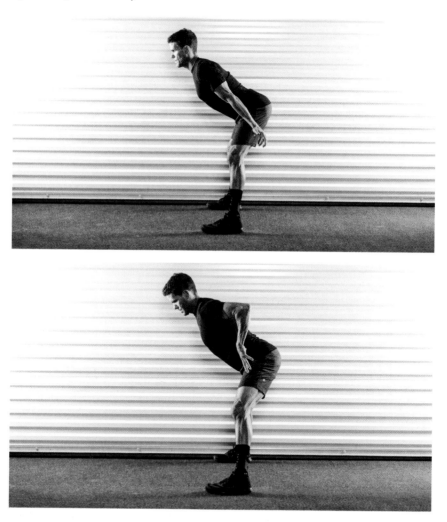

Touch your thumbs to your hips. Now trace them up your sides, keeping your elbows as high as possible, past your lats, the back of your head, and to full extension. Now trace back the way you came. Brace again for the next rep.

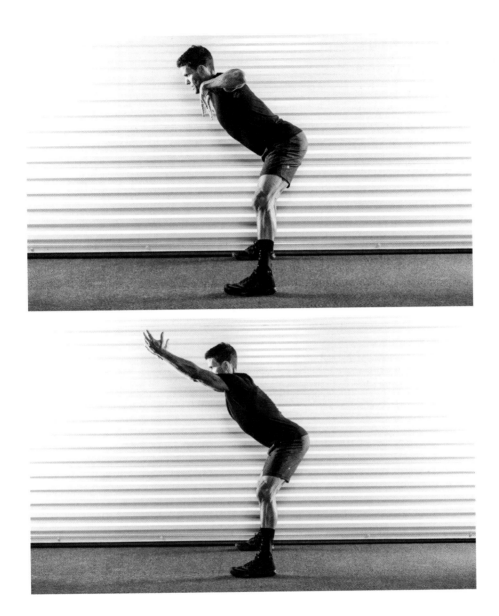

> WIDE FOUNDER WITH GORILLA REACH

Gorilla reach is another wide founder progression that helps you regain shoulder mobility and gets you activated for your workout.

Put a kettlebell or any short object in front of you. Get into a wide founder position. Reach out with one hand, with your thumb pointed out so your shoulders stay packed. Take a sniff of air, and brace your abs. Now, reach up, then come back down and alternate with the other arm.

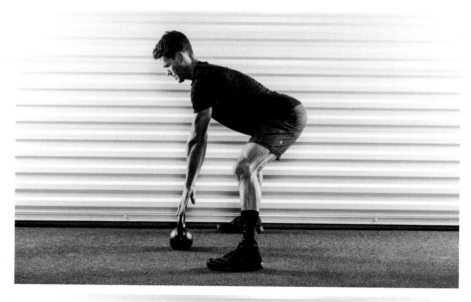

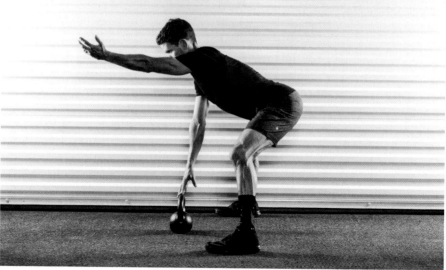

> GOBLET SQUAT HOLDS

Some years back I started dedicating a few hours in the afternoon to increasing my flexibility, getting deep into my tight tissue, strengthening my core, while listening to loud music. Pretty soon some of the other trainers at Platinum joined me, and then some of my clients, and what evolved over time has now become a twice-weekly class in which friends, trainers, and athletes come to foam roll, smash, stretch, and do ab work and lots of Foundation movements—and of course, listen to loud music. At the end of the session, much to a lot of peoples' chagrin, we finish with a goblet squat hold. At first we just did one-minute holds, but over the years, well, you know how things progress. We're up to five minutes now.

Is this some kind of test or torture? No. Okay, sorta. Sometimes cocky athletes come to class, and it's fun to watch them squirm trying to squat low for five minutes. But there's true purpose to a squat hold too: I find most peoples' adductors, ankles, and hips loosen up the longer they can hold a weighted goblet squat. In East Beach you'll just hold the position for one minute. But just as in my class, things progress, and we'll keep adding time—thirty seconds here, another minute there—until you hit the magic number in the final workout: the five-minute goblet squat. The biggest challenge is maintaining your posture. If you do default, stand up, refocus, rebrace, and start again. Here are your cues.

Using a lighter weight, bring the kettlebell or dumbbell to your chest. Start creating tension, take a breath, brace the abs, and then drop slowly down into a deep squat. Be sure to keep your heels on the ground, your back flat, your shoulders back, and your chin neutral. As you hold your position, use your elbows to push out your knees and try to sink lower. Lastly, play some tunes good and loud, and oh how time will fly!

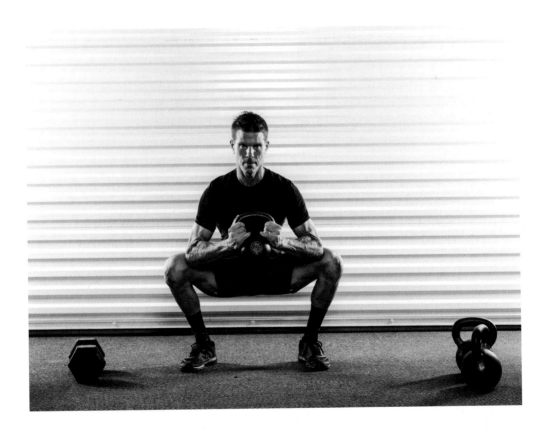

Activation—1x

Ankle Mobility	Bird Dogs	T-Spine Rotations	Body Weight Squat	Hip Hinge	Knee Drop	Woodpecker
10 pulses outward, middle and inward for each ankle ➤	10x alternating sides ➤	10x per side ➤	10x ➤	10x ➤	10x per side ➤	• 15-second holds • 10 hinges • 10 rotations, per side

Core Round—2x

Oblique Roll	Eight-Point Plank
7x per side ➤	15-second holds, 10-second rest, 15-second holds with knees off the ground

Circuit One—2x

Goblet Squat	Pushups	Farmer Carries	Pushups
10x ➤	Go until one before failure ➤	30-second walk ➤	Go until one before failure

Circuit Two—2x

Romanian Dead Lift	Bench Rows	Getups: Punch-Up to Elbow
10x ➤	10x per side ➤	5x per side

Cardio

Warm Up	Main Set	Cool Down
1 minute easy, 2x 30-seconds at 80% effort, with 30 seconds off between sets ➤	• 5x 20 seconds at 80% effort, 40 seconds slow between sets • 5x 20 seconds at 85% effort, 40 seconds slow between sets ➤	Go easy for two minutes

Recovery

Couch Stretch	T-Spine Smash
2 minutes per side ➤	4 minutes

MOVEMENT PRACTICE: Circuit One—1x

Ankle Mobility	Bird Dogs	T-Spine Rotations	Founder	Hip Hinge
10 pulses outward, middle and inward for each ankle ➤	10x alternating sides ➤	10x per side ➤	2x 15-second holds, 10-second rest between sets ➤	12x ➤

Circuit Two—1x

Lunge Stretch + Knee Drops	Woodpecker	Body Weight Squat	Wide Founder
2x 10-second holds, 7x knee drops, 10-second rest, per side ➤	• 15-second holds • 10x hinges • 10 rotations, per side	12x ➤	3x 15-second holds (focus on creating full-body tension), 10-second rest between sets

Core Round—2x

Oblique Roll	Eight-Point Plank
7x per side ➤	15-second holds, 10-second rest, 15-second holds with knees off the ground, 10-second rest

Cardio

30 minutes of low-intensity, base-building cardio at 60–70% exertion.

Recovery

Psoas Smash	Glute/TFL Smash
2 minutes per side ➤	2 minutes per side, rolling slowly over tight spots

Activation—1x

Ankle Mobility	Bird Dogs	T-Spine Rotations	Body Weight Squat	Hip Hinge	Knee Drop	Woodpecker
10 pulses outward, middle and inward for each ankle ➤	10x alternating sides ➤	10x per side ➤	10x ➤	10x ➤	10x per side ➤	• 15-second holds • 10 hinges • 10 rotations, per side

Core Round—2x

Eight-Point Plank	Side Plank
15-second holds, 10-second rest, 15-second holds with knees off the ground, 10-second rest ➤	3x 10-second hold per side, 10-second rest between sets

Circuit One—2x

Goblet Squat	Pushups	Farmer Carries	Pushups
10x ➤	Go until one before failure ➤	30-second walk ➤	Go until one before failure

Circuit Two—2x

Romanian Dead Lift	Bench Rows	Getups: Punch-Up to Elbow
10x ➤	10x per side ➤	5x per side

Cardio

Warm Up	Main Set	Cool Down
1 minute easy, 2x 30-seconds at 80% effort, with 30 seconds off between sets ➤	6x 30-second intervals, at 80% effort, increasing to 85%, 1 minute recovery pace between sets ➤	Go easy for two minutes

Recovery

Pec Smash	Hamstring Smash
2 minutes per side ➤	2 minutes per leg

Activation—1x

Ankle Mobility	Bird Dogs	T-Spine Rotations	Body Weight Squat	Hip Hinge	Knee Drop	Woodpecker
10 pulses outward, middle and inward for each ankle ➤	10x alternating sides ➤	10x per side ➤	12x ➤	12x ➤	10, per side ➤	• 10 hinges • 10 rotations, per side

Core Round—2x

Oblique Roll	Eight-Point Plank
10x per side ➤	15-second holds, 10-second rest, 15-second holds with knees off the ground, 10-second rest between sets

Circuit One—3x

Goblet Squat	Pushups	Farmer Carries	Pushups
10x, pull yourself down slowly into the squat ➤	Go until one before failure ➤	30-second walk ➤	Go until one before failure

Circuit Two—3x

Romanian Dead Lift	Bench Rows	Getups: Punch-Up Kneeling Lunge
10x knees back, back flat ➤	10x per side ➤	2x per side

Cardio

Warm Up	Main Set	Cool Down
1 minute easy, 2x 30-seconds at 80% effort, with 30 seconds off between sets ➤	5x 1-minute at 80% effort, 1-minute easy pace between sets ➤	Go easy for two minutes

Recovery

Diaphragm Smash	Hamstring Smash
4 minutes ➤	2 minutes per leg

MOVEMENT PRACTICE: Circuit One—1x

Ankle Mobility	Bird Dogs	T-Spine Rotations	Founder	Hip Hinge
10 pulses outward, middle and inward for each ankle ➤	10x alternating sides ➤	10x per side ➤	3x 15-second holds, 10-second rest between sets ➤	15x

Circuit Two—1x

Lunge Stretch + Knee Drops	Woodpecker	Body Weight Squat	Wide Founder + Gorilla Reaches
1x 15-second holds, 10x knee drops, per side ➤	• 15-second holds • 10 hinges • 10 rotations, per side	12x ➤	• 2x 15-second Wide Founder holds • 7x Gorilla Reaches, per side

Core Round—2x

Oblique Roll	Eight-Point Plank
7x per side ➤	15-second holds, 10-second rest, 15-second holds with knees off the ground, 10-second rest

Cardio

30 minutes of low-intensity, base-building cardio at 60–70% exertion.
Optional: pick three machines, do 5 minutes per machine 2x

Recovery

Pigeon Stretch	Lat-to-Rotator Roll
2 minutes per side, remember to breathe to go deeper into the stretch ➤	2 minutes per side, rolling slowly over tight spots

Activation—1x

Ankle Mobility	Bird Dogs	T-Spine Rotations	Body Weight Squat	Hip Hinge	Knee Drop	Woodpecker
10 pulses outward, middle and inward for each ankle ➤	10x alternating sides ➤	10x per side ➤	12x ➤	12x ➤	10x per side ➤	• 10 hinges • 10 rotations, per side

Core Round—2x

Side Plank	Eight-Point Plank
2x 15-second holds, per side ➤	3x 15-second holds with knees off the ground, 10-second rest

Circuit One—3x

Goblet Squat	Pushups	Farmer Carries	Pushups
10x, take it slow on the way down, then power up ➤	Go until one before failure ➤	30-second walk ➤	Go until one before failure

Circuit Two—3x

Romanian Dead Lift	Bench Rows	Getups: Punch-Up to Kneeling Lunge
10x, focusing on creating tension ➤	10x per side ➤	2x per side

Cardio

Warm Up	Main Set	Cool Down
1 minute easy, 2x 30-seconds at 80% effort, with 30 seconds off between sets ➤	5x 45 seconds at 80% effort, 15 seconds recover pace between intervals, 2 minute rest, repeat ➤	Go easy for two minutes

Recovery

Adductor Stretch	Calf Smash
2 minutes per side ➤	2 minutes per leg

Activation—1x

Ankle Mobility	Bird Dogs	T-Spine Rotations	Body Weight Squat	Hip Hinge	Knee Drop	Woodpecker
10 pulses outward, middle and inward for each ankle ➤	10x alternating sides ➤	10x per side ➤	10x ➤	10x ➤	10x per side ➤	• 10 hinges • 10 rotations, per side

Core Round—2x

Eight-Point Plank	Side Plank
3x 15-second holds with knees off the ground, 10-second rest between holds ➤	2x 15-second holds per side, 10-second rest between sets

Circuit One—3x
(The reps in this week's circuits drop from 10 to 8, so try to increase your weight.)

Goblet Squat	Pushups	Farmer Carries	Pushups
8x, heels remain flat on the floor ➤	Go until one before failure ➤	30-second walk, heavier weight ➤	Go until one before failure

Circuit Two—3x

Romanian Dead Lift	Bench Rows	Full Getups
8x, squeeze glutes, brace core tight ➤	10x per side ➤	2x per side

Cardio

Warm Up	Main Set	Cool Down
1 minute easy, 2x 30-seconds at 80% effort, with 30 seconds off between sets ➤	• 2 minutes at 70–80% effort, then 2 minutes at recovery pace • 2x 1-minute at 85% effort, 1 minute at recovery pace between • 3x 30-second intervals at 80-85% effort, 1 minute recovery pace between intervals ➤	Go easy for two minutes

Recovery

Couch Stretch	T-Spine Smash
2 minutes per side ➤	4 minutes

MOVEMENT PRACTICE: Circuit One—1x

Ankle Mobility	Bird Dogs	T-Spine Rotations	Founder	Hip Hinge
10 pulses outward, middle and inward for each ankle ➤	10x alternating sides ➤	10x per side ➤	3x 15-second holds, 10-second rest between sets ➤	12x

Circuit Two—1x

Lunge Stretch + Knee Drops	Woodpecker	Body Weight Squat	Wide Founder + Gorilla Reaches
1x 15-second holds, 10x knee drops, per side ➤	• 15-second holds • 10 hinges • 10 rotations, per side	12x ➤	• 15-second Wide Founder hold • 7x Gorilla Reaches, per side

Core Round—1x

Oblique Roll	Eight-Point Plank
7x per side ➤	3x 15-second holds with knees off the ground, 10-second rest between holds

Cardio

30 minutes of low-intensity, base-building cardio at 60–70% exertion.
Optional: pick three machines, do 10 minutes each

Recovery

Psoas Smash	Glute/TFL Smash
2 minutes per side ➤	2 minutes per side, rolling slowly over tight spots

Activation—1x

Ankle Mobility	Bird Dogs	T-Spine Rotations	Body Weight Squat	Hip Hinge	Knee Drop	Woodpecker
10 pulses outward, middle and inward for each ankle ➤	10x alternating sides ➤	10x per side ➤	10x ➤	10x ➤	10x per side ➤	• 10 hinges • 10 rotations, per side

Core Round—2x

Eight-Point Plank

3x 15-second holds, knees off the ground, 10-second rest between holds ➤

Side Plank

2x 15-second holds per side, 10-second rest between

Circuit One—3x

Goblet Squat

8x ➤

Pushups

Go until one before failure ➤

Farmer Carries

30-second walk ➤

Pushups

Go until one before failure

Circuit Two—3x

Romanian Dead Lift

8x ➤

Bench Rows

8x per side ➤

Full Getups

2x per side

Cardio

Warm Up

1 minute easy, 2x 30-seconds at 80% effort, with 30 seconds off between sets ➤

Main Set

3 x 3 minutes at 80% effort, 2 minutes recovery pace between ➤

Cool Down

Go easy for two minutes

Recovery

Pec Smash

2 minutes per pec ➤

Hamstring Smash

2 minutes per leg

Circuit One—1x

Founder

3x 15-second holds,
10-second rest between ➤

Hip Hinge

12x ➤

Lunge Stretch + Knee Drop

2x 10-second holds, then
7x knee drops, per side

Circuit Two—1x

Wide Founder with Tracing + Hold + Gorilla Reaches

• 7x Traces
• 10-second holds
• 10x Gorilla Reaches
  alternating arms ➤

Body Weight Squat

12x ➤

Woodpecker

• 15-second holds
• 10 hinges
• 10 rotations, per side

Circuit Three—1x

Bird Dogs

10x alternating sides
➤

T-Spine Rotations

10x per side ➤

Eight-Point Plank

3x 15-second holds with
knees off the ground,
10-second rest between
holds ➤

Pushups

Go until one before
failure

Core Round—2x

Oblique Roll

7x per side ➤

Side Plank

2x 15-second holds per side, 10-second rest
between

Goblet Squat Hold—60 seconds

Cardio

30 minutes of easy, low-intensity cardio at 60–70% exertion.

Recovery

Hamstring Stretch

2 minutes per side ➤

Diaphragm Smash

4 minutes

EAST BEACH: WEEK FOUR ➤ DAY TWO

STRENGTH MAINTENANCE: Activation—1x

Ankle Mobility	Bird Dogs	T-Spine Rotations	Knee Drop	Woodpecker	Body Weight Squat	Hip Hinge
10 pulses outward, middle and inward for each ankle ➤	10x alternating sides ➤	10x per side ➤	10x per side ➤	• 1x 10-second holds • 10 hinges • 10 rotations, per side ➤	12x ➤	12x (go slow, keep your chest forward)

Core Round—2x

Eight-Point Plank
3x 15-second holds with knees off the ground, 10-second rest between holds ➤

Side Plank
12x 15-second holds, alternating sides

Circuit One—2x

Goblet Squat
8x, pull yourself down slowly to bottom of squat, hold one second, power back up ➤

Pushups
Go until one before failure ➤

Farmer Carries
30-second walk, increase weight ➤

Pushups
Go until one before failure

Cardio

Warm Up
1 minute easy, 2x 30-seconds at 80% effort, with 30 seconds off between sets ➤

Main Set
• 4x 10-second sprints at 90–95% effort, 30 seconds between sprints
• 2 minutes rest between sets ➤

Cool Down
Go easy for two minutes

Recovery

Lat-to-Rotator Cuff Roll
2 minutes per side ➤

Pigeon Stretch
2 minutes per side

Circuit One—1x

Founder
3x 15-second holds,
10-second rest between ➤

Hip Hinge
12x ➤

Lunge Stretch + Knee Drop
2x 10-second holds, then
7x knee drops, per side

Circuit Two—1x

Wide Founder with Tracing + Hold + Gorilla Reaches
• 7x Traces
• 10-second holds
• 10x Gorilla Reaches
  alternating arms ➤

Body Weight Squat
12x ➤

Woodpecker
• 15-second holds
• 10 hinges
• 10 rotations, per side

Circuit Three—1x

Bird Dogs
10x alternating sides
➤

T-Spine Rotations
10x per side ➤

Eight-Point Plank
3x 15-second holds with
knees off the ground,
10-second rest between
holds ➤

Pushups
Go until one before
failure

Core Round—2x

Oblique Roll
7x per side ➤

Side Plank
2x 15-second holds per side, 10-second rest
between

Goblet Squat Hold—60 seconds

Cardio

30 minutes of easy, low-intensity cardio at 60–70% exertion.
Optional: Choose three machines and go 5 minutes on each , 2x

Recovery

Adductor Stretch
2 minutes per side ➤

Calf Smash
2 minutes per side, rolling slowly
over tight spots

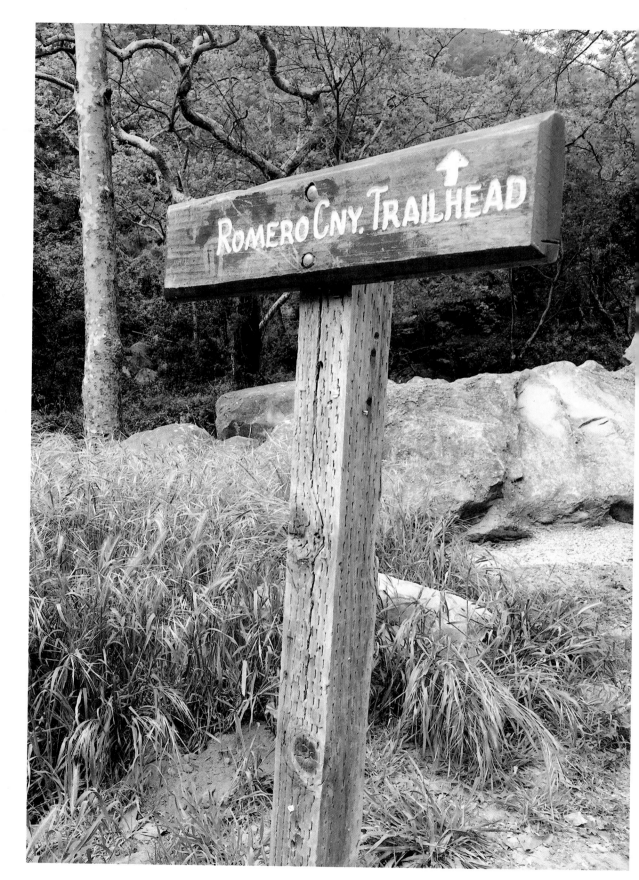

CHAPTER NINE: ROMERO CANYON

WHENEVER LANCE ARMSTRONG CAME TO Santa Barbara to train with me, the first order of business was a mountain bike ride up Romero Canyon. We'd ride from the trailhead up the fire road to the top of the mountain, then race back down like kids. It was so much fun that we'd turn around and ride right back up again, trying to beat our previous time. Typically the round trip took about seventy-five minutes. Back at the bottom again we'd ditch our bikes, then race up the single-track trail on foot, turn around at the top, and speed down the desolate fire road to the bottom. Then, we'd race back up to beat our time (hopefully) before heading back down again. Those were the days. Every birthday I still race up Romero on my bike with the goal of beating my own age. Last year I turned fifty-two, and I did it in forty-seven minutes. Can't wait to turn seventy!

In the Romero Canyon workout you'll start using a kettlebell while doing your getup, and you'll also learn another kettlebell exercise called swings. Swings are an explosive exercise and in a class unto themselves. Like the getup, they're complex and take time to get just right, but once you master them, you'll have a workout partner for life.

In week one you're going to do a cardio time trial to establish a baseline measure of your cardio fitness level. Then for the next two weeks we raise the intensity of your cardio workouts, and test you again at the end of week four to check your progress. Hope you enjoy Romero Canyon as much as Lance and I used to. It's a good one.

NEW EXERCISES

> GLUTE BRIDGES

PROPS: You'll need a foam roller or a pillow.

Do you have glute amnesia? Then let these bridges help your glutes remember they exist. No other activation exercise fires up the glutes and hamstrings better than bridges. In this activation movement you'll lift your back up and then reach your arms back to get a shoulder stretch—a twofer.

Start by lying on your back with your feet flat on the floor about six inches apart and knees bent at 90 degrees. Your arms should be at your side. Put the foam roller between your knees. Now, start digging your elbows into the floor, squeeze your glutes, brace your abs, and dig your heels into the floor. Drive your hips up to full extension without hyperextending your back, while squeezing the roller and your glutes together as tightly as you can. Focus on isolating your glutes to power the bridge.

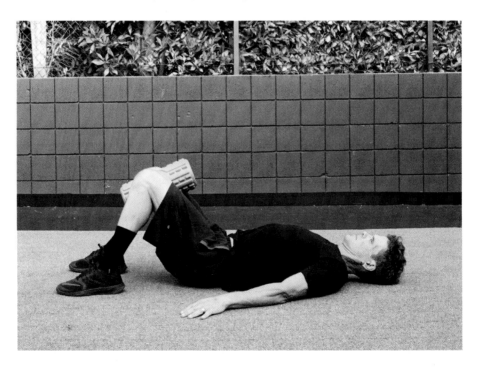

At the top of your bridge, extend your arms above you, and create a sphere of tension. While keeping arms extended, pack your shoulders down and slowly bring your arms back toward the floor as far as you can until you feel a good stretch in your back and lats.

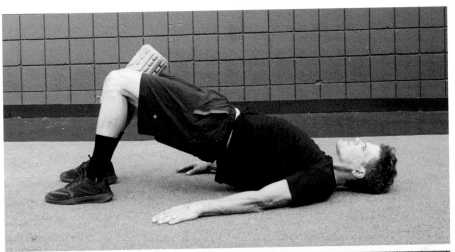

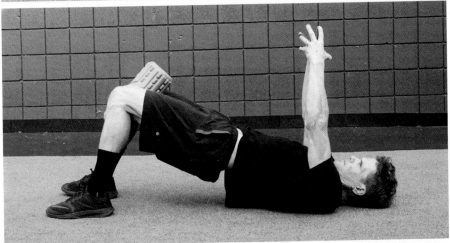

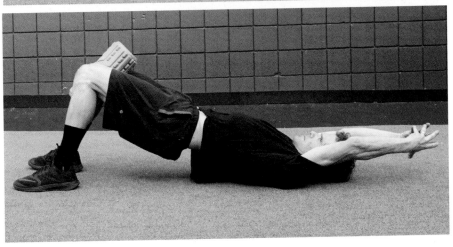

> SINGLE-ARM FLOOR PRESS

Single-arm floor presses are a safer and a more controlled way of working the chest, lats, shoulders, and triceps. A lot of people with shoulder pain who can't do a bench press or even a pushup find they can do floor presses. As an added bonus, pressing one arm at a time forces you to stabilize your core, which can help correct imbalances. (Often you'll notice one side of your body is much more stable than the other.) Like a bench press, you'll feel your pectoral muscles and the shoulders doing much of the work, but by creating tension through your core and lats, the whole upper body and your core get worked. Keep the movement under control at all times, especially as you lower the weight.

Start on the floor in the fetal position, holding the kettlebell or dumbbell in the bottom (left) hand. Roll onto your back, bringing the weight up, extending your arm so the weight is directly above you. Drop your right hand to the floor. Your feet should be shoulder-width apart and your arm in a neutral position. If using a kettlebell, your thumb's on top of it, as if holding a hammer.

Now pack your shoulders into the floor, take in a sniff, and brace your abs as you lift your opposite (right) leg six inches off the floor and hold it there. Take another sniff of air, brace again, and slowly row the weight down, focusing on pulling with your lats, until your elbow touches the floor. Rebrace your body, then drive the weight back up, keeping your shoulders pressed in the floor.

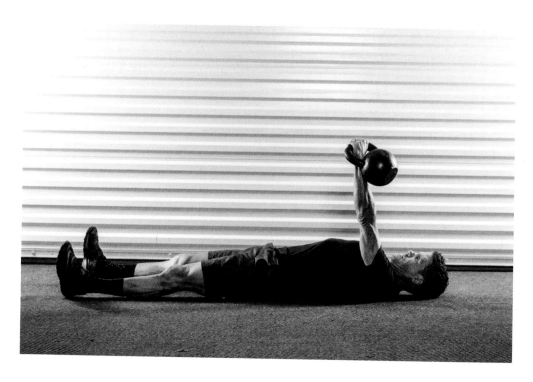

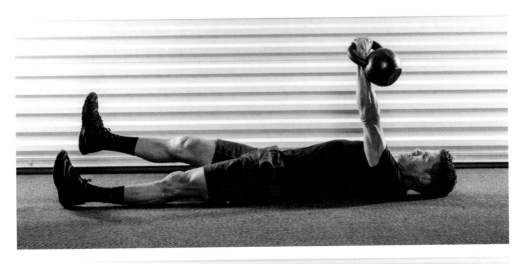

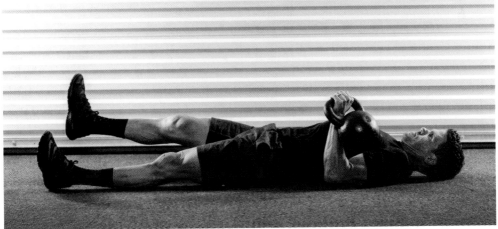

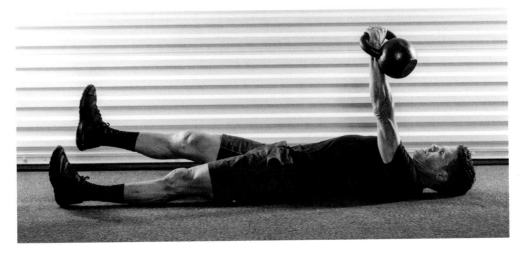

> HIP HINGE ROWS

In East Beach you learned how to do Romanian dead lifts. The hip hinge row adds a rowing component to RDLs. In this exercise you kill two birds with one stone: you work the posterior chain at the same time as you're working your lats and upper back during the row.

Get into the bottom position of the RDL with two kettlebells or dumbbells. Starting with arms extended and shoulders packed down and lats locked, begin rowing the weights up, keeping your elbows at 90 degrees. Keep pulling the weights up to your end point. Your body should remain in a perfect hinge position with hips back, back flat, posture perfect.

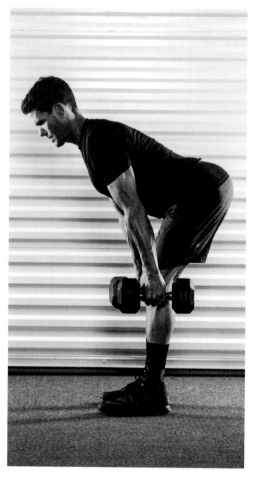 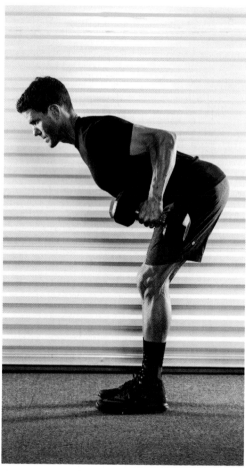

> BULGARIAN SPLIT SQUATS

Bulgarian split squats are one of the best exercises you can do to build glute, hip, and quad strength. Why work one leg at a time? Many of us become stronger (or weaker) in one leg (and arm and glute) over the years. Working each leg separately corrects those weaknesses and improves whole-body balance by fixing right-to-left discrepancies. (Same can be said of most one-leg or one-arm exercises.) Bulgarians will also stabilize supporting muscles in the hips, and are a great way to load the muscles with minimal stress on the spine.

Holding weights in both hands, stand in a split stance with a bench behind you. Put one foot in front of you and the other on the bench behind you, shoelaces facing down. Move your front foot far enough forward so that the knee is directly over the ankle and back foot is on the edge of the bench. Take a sniff of air, brace your abs, and lock in.

Now, slowly drop your back knee until you're about an inch from the floor, then drive up, pushing through the midfoot. Make sure your torso remains upright or slightly leaning forward. Keep good posture throughout the entire range of motion. Rebrace and drive back up to starting position.

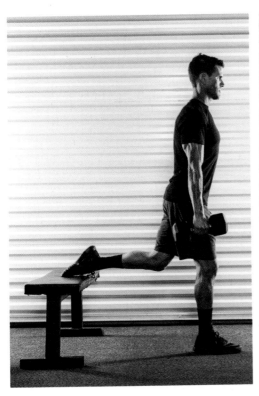
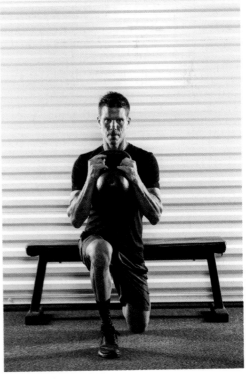

> KETTLEBELL SWINGS

Kettlebell swings run a tight race with getups as the single-most effective exercise. And although they're easy to learn, like a baseball or golf swing, they're difficult to master.

What makes them so effective? First, swings are a dynamic exercise that build power and cardio endurance, all the while working your glutes, hamstrings, abs, shoulders, and grip strength. And because you do them with an explosive movement, a big hip thrust forward, swings increase power, build coordination and core stability, and improve your movement patterns. Convinced?

There are two distinct movements to kettlebell swings that are linked together. The first is an explosive hip thrust that propels the weight upward and outward in front of you. The second movement is pulling the weight back down between your legs before thrusting it back up again.

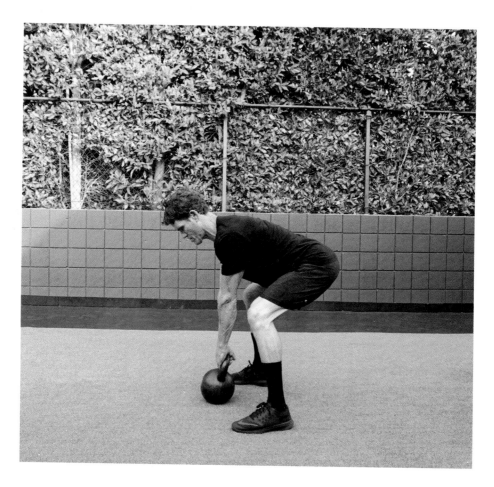

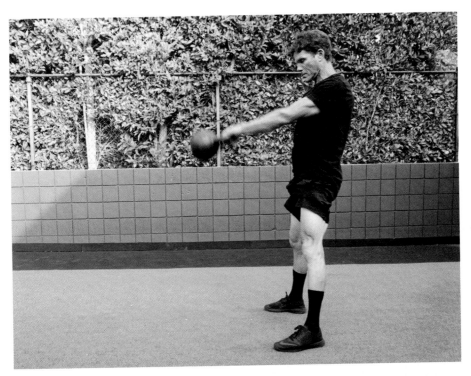

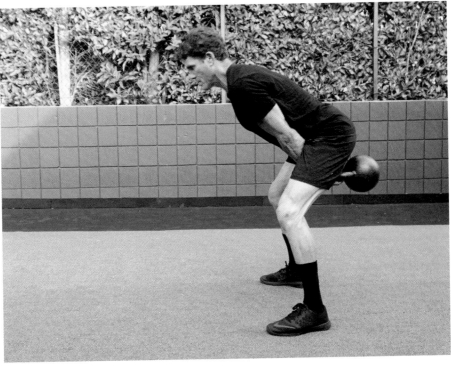

Most of the people I train pick up the basic technique of swings in just a few weeks, but as with the Turkish getup, I've divided swings into phases, each taught over the course of a week. Phase one is called behind-the-back kettlebell hinges, which will now become a mainstay of your activation routine.

> BEHIND-THE-BACK KETTLEBELL HINGES

You've already learned how to hinge, and now, by adding a kettlebell behind you to the movement, you'll reinforce the pattern and force yourself to pull back your shoulders and lock your upper back.

Start with your feet about shoulder-width apart. Grab a kettlebell by the horns, and position it behind your back, holding it with both hands. Actively pull your shoulders down and lock your lats. Squeeze your glutes. Take a sniff in, and brace your abs.

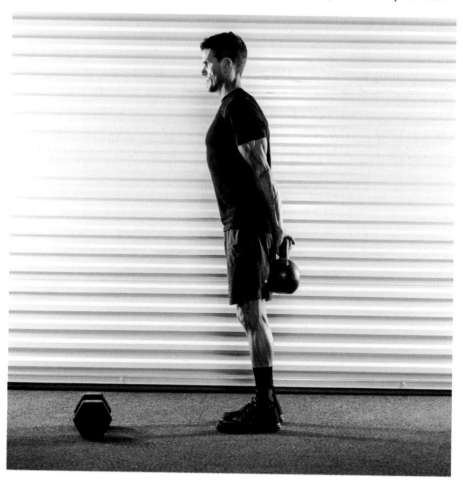

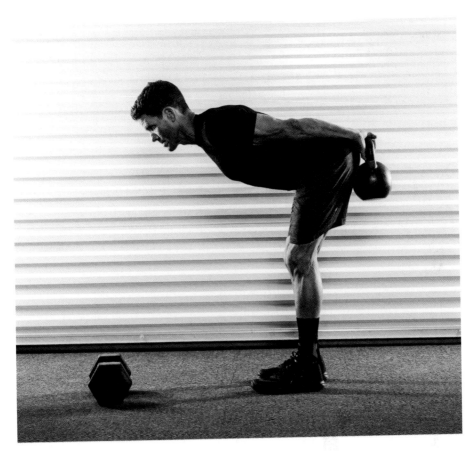

Drive your hips backward as if pushing a drawer behind you closed while pushing your chest forward. Keep pushing your hips back until you feel a stretch in the hamstrings and glutes. Make sure to keep your knees slightly bent as you descend to the bottom of the hinge. At the bottom brace again, and with a powerful but controlled hip drive, return to the starting position.

> KETTLEBELL DEAD LIFTS

In East Beach you learned Romanian dead lifts with two weights. Kettlebell dead lifts with just one weight is a progression that helps you to do swings.

Start with your feet a little more than shoulder-width apart and your toes pointed slightly outward. The weight should be positioned at your midfoot. Slowly hinge your hips back, keeping your back as flat as possible. Grab the kettlebell, keeping your arms extended and looking slightly forward. If your back starts to round, try elevating the weight six inches or a foot.

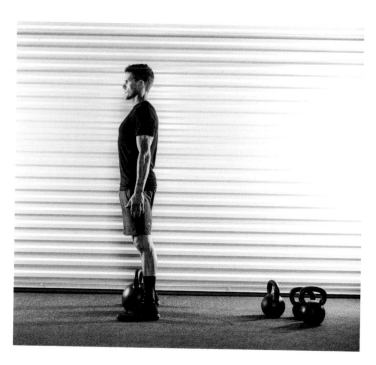

Create tension by gripping the horns as though you are trying to break them apart. Pull your shoulders down, and lock your lats. Take a sniff of air, and brace your abs.

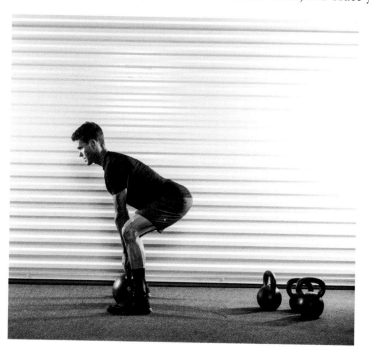

Squeeze your glutes, and drive the kettlebell up, using a powerful hip thrust. At the top position abs are tight, glutes squeezed, core braced. Maintaining that perfect hinge pattern, slowly return the weights to the floor. Rebrace for the next rep.

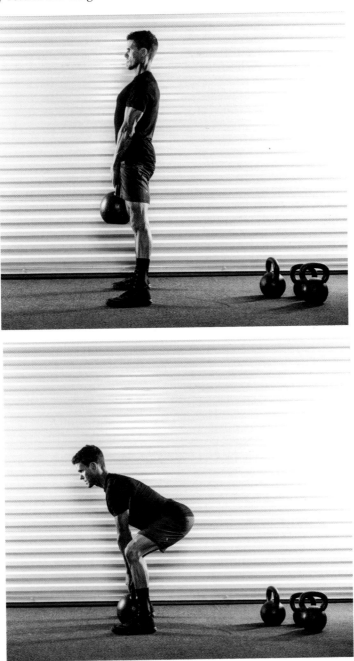

> *TURKISH GETUP WITH KETTLEBELL*

In the East Beach workout you learned how to do the getup with a mock weight (page 122). Now it's time to use the real thing, a kettlebell. Gripping the kettlebell properly during during the movement is important. Make sure your wrist is locked straight (don't let it bend backwards.) Also important, your elbow needs to be locked and your shoulders packed down (no shrugging allowed.) Try to move at a slow and controlled pace. Lastly, keep your eyes on the kettlebell (it's safer) until you've reached the kneeling position.

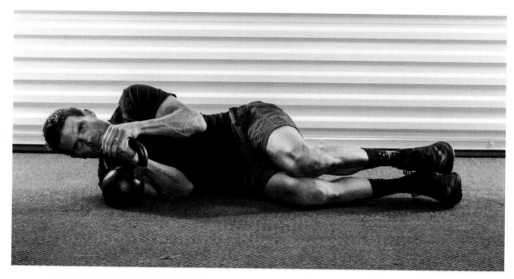

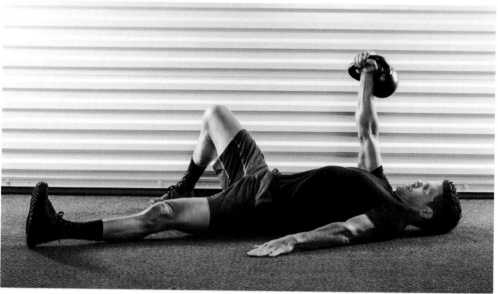

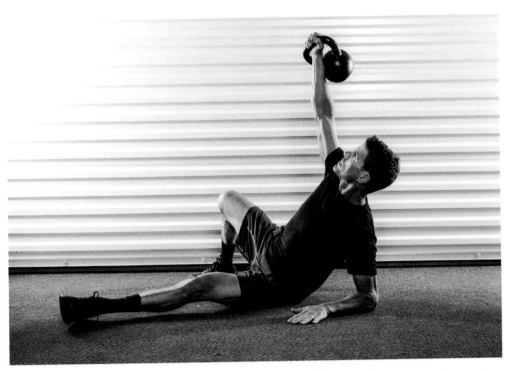

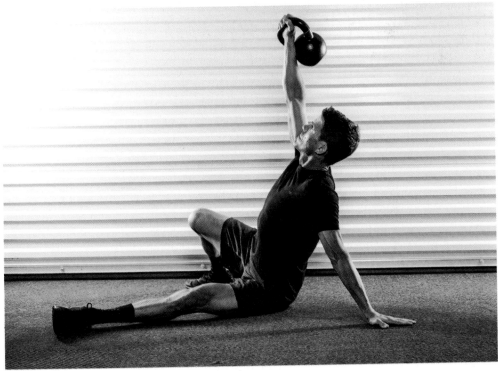

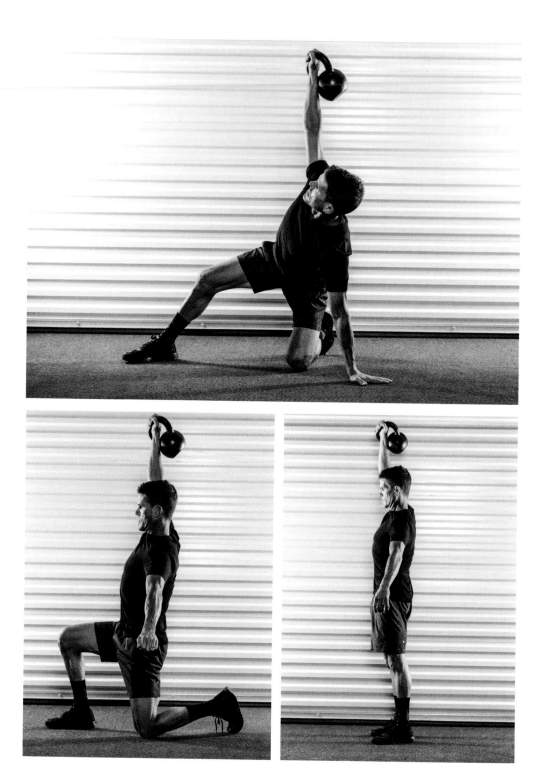

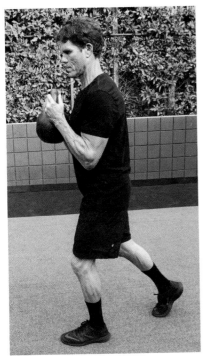

> GOBLET SQUAT CARRIES

This is an irresistible mashup featuring the best aspects of two great exercises, goblet squats and farmer carries. As you learned on page 117, in goblet squats you frontload the body, forcing your abs to brace to lend lower back support which gives them a workout. You're also getting a good cardio workout by taking a stroll while holding weight.

To do goblet squat carries, hinge over, brace, and lift the weight to your chest. Brace your abs, check your posture, and then take a stroll for the directed amount of time. Make sure your posture stays strong throughout.

> ROLLOUTS ON STABILITY BALL

Rollouts on the stability ball teach your body to stabilize during dynamic rolling motion. And that dynamic motion for this core exercise is drawing the alphabet with your arms as you balance on the ball, trying to remain stable in an unstable position.

Put your feet against a wall, the stability ball in front of you. Now get into an eight-point plank position on the ball, with your knees bent at 90 degrees, about six inches off the floor. With your elbows on the ball and your arms bent at 90 degrees, take a sniff of air, and brace the abs. Now start "drawing" the alphabet slowly, using big movements. (The first week you'll write out the alphabet A through L, the second week M through Z, and the last week you'll do the whole alphabet.) Want to add a mental challenge? Do the alphabet backward.

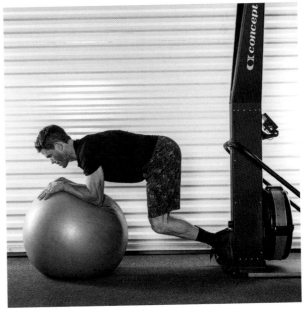

> KETTLEBELL SWINGS

You already know how to do a kettlebell swing. You just don't know it. The kettlebell hinge in Week One and the kettlebell dead lift in Week Two taught you the important steps. What's left comes in Week Three: hiking the kettlebell and exploding up with it.

Start with your feet a little more than shoulder-width apart, your toes slightly pointed out, and your arms reaching out in front of you, grabbing onto the kettlebell handle. Get your back flat and your hips pushed back, your shoulders packed down, and your shins vertical. Take a breath, and brace your core.

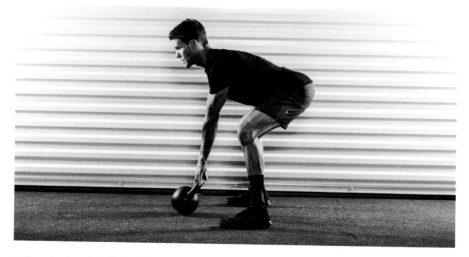

Drive the kettlebell back between your legs until your forearms make contact with your inner thighs, like you're about to hike a football. This should happen in a single, swift movement.

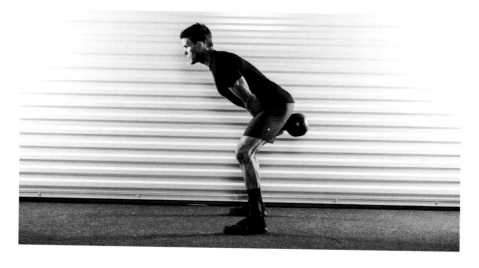

Now, explosively drive your hips forward, swinging the kettlebell up. As you go, focus on driving the kettlebell with your hips (not lifting it with your arms). Keep your shoulders packed down and core braced. At the top of the movement—in a millisecond pause—the kettlebell should feel weightless. Take the opportunity here to squeeze your quads, butt, and rebrace your abs.

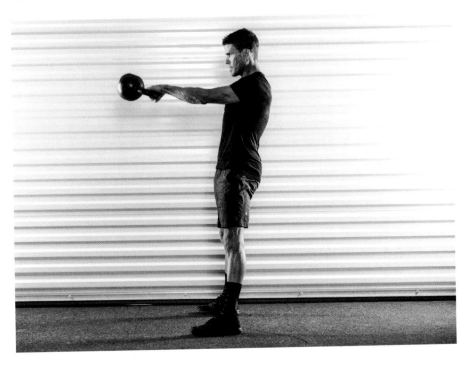

Pull the kettlebell back down, guiding it between your legs and as close to the groin as possible for the next rep. Remember, the kettlebell swing is a hinge movement, not a squat. There's no rest between reps. You want to establish a swift rhythm like other dynamic exercises. A hip thrust up, a pull back down. Inhale on the way up through your nose and exhale at the top of your teeth.

Activation—1x

Ankle Mobility	Bird Dogs	T-Spine Rotations	Glute Bridges	Goblet Squat	Behind the Back Hinge
10 pulses outward, middle and inward for each ankle ➤	10x alternating sides ➤	10x per side ➤	10x bridges, 10x extensions ➤	10x ➤	10x

Core Round—2x

Roll-Outs on Stability Ball	Janda Crunch
Draw the alphabet A–L ➤	7x

Circuit One—2x

Hinge Row	Bulgarian Split Squat	Goblet Squat Walk
10x ➤	10x per side ➤	30-second walk

Circuit Two—2x

Single-arm Floor Press	Kettlebell Dead Lifts	Getups with Weight
10x per side ➤	10x ➤	1x per side, keep your eye locked on the kettlebell until lunge position

Cardio

Time Trial: A time trial measures the amount of time it takes you to cover a given distance, on the bike, treadmill, or whatever machine you choose. Stick with the same machine for all of Romero Canyon and we'll test you again.

Warm Up: 1 minute easy, 2x 30-seconds at 80% effort with 30 seconds off between sets.

Time Trial: Choose one fo the following cardio machines:

- **Stationary bike:** Pedal 3 miles
- **Rower or skier:** 2000 meters
- **Treadmill:** 1.5 miles
- **Elliptical:** 1.5 miles
- **Versa Climber:** 1,500 feet

Cool Down: Go easy for two minutes

Recovery

Couch Stretch	T-Spine Smash
2 minutes per side ➤	4 minutes

MOVEMENT PRACTICE: Circuit One—1x

Founder

3x 15-second holds, 10-second rest between ➤

Hip Hinge

12x ➤

Lunge Stretch + Knee Drop

15-second holds, 10 knee drops, per side

Circuit Two—1x

Wide Founder with Tracing + Hold + Gorilla Reaches

- 7x Traces
- 10-second holds
- 10x Gorilla Reaches alternating arms ➤

Body Weight Squat

12x ➤

Woodpecker

- 15-second holds
- 10 hinges
- 10 rotations, per side

Circuit Three—1x

Bird Dogs

10x alternating sides ➤

T-Spine Rotations

10x per side ➤

Eight-Point Plank

3x 15-second holds with knees off the ground, 10-second rest between holds ➤

Pushups

5x 5 pushups, 20-second rest in between all 5 sets

Core Round—1x

Roll-Outs on Stability Ball

Draw the alphabet A–L ➤

Janda Crunch

7x ➤

Side Plank

3x 30-second hold per side, 10-second rest between

Goblet Squat Hold—2 minutes

Cardio

30 minutes of low-intensity, base-building cardio at 60–70% exertion.

Recovery

Psoas Smash

2 minutes per side ➤

Glute/TFL Smash

2 minutes per side, rolling slowly over tight spots.

Activation—1x

Ankle Mobility	Bird Dogs	T-Spine Rotations	Glute Bridges	Goblet Squat	Behind the Back Hinge
10 pulses outward, middle and inward for each ankle ➤	10x alternating sides ➤	10x per side ➤	10x bridges, 10x extensions ➤	10x ➤	10x

Core Round—2x

Roll-Outs on Stability Ball	Janda Crunch
Draw the alphabet A–L ➤	7x

Circuit One—2x

Hinge Row	Bulgarian Split Squat	Goblet Squat Walk
10x ➤	10x per side ➤	30-second walk

Circuit Two—2x

Single-arm Floor Press	Kettlebell Dead Lifts	Getups with Weight
10x per side ➤	10x ➤	1x per side, keep your eye locked on the kettlebell until lunge position

Cardio

Warm Up	Main Set	Cool Down
1 minute easy, 2x 30-seconds at 80% effort, with 30 seconds off between sets ➤	• 5x 1 minute at 85–90% effort, 2 minutes recovery pace between ➤	Go easy for two minutes

Recovery

Pec Smash	Hamstring Smash
2 minutes per pec ➤	2 minutes per leg

Activation—1x

Ankle Mobility	Bird Dogs	T-Spine Rotations	Glute Bridges	Goblet Squat	Behind the Back Hinge
10 pulses outward, middle and inward for each ankle ➤	10x alternating sides ➤	10x per side ➤	10x bridges, 10x extensions ➤	10x ➤	10x

Core Round—2x

Roll-Outs on Stability Ball	Janda Crunch
Draw the alphabet M–Z ➤	7x

Circuit One—2x

Hinge Row	Bulgarian Split Squat	Goblet Squat Walk
10x ➤	10x per side ➤	30-second walk

Circuit Two—2x

Single-arm Floor Press	Kettlebell Dead Lifts	Getups with Weight
10x per side ➤	10x ➤	1x per side, keep your eye locked on the kettlebell until lunge position

Cardio

Warm Up: 1 minute easy, 2x 30-seconds at 80% effort with 30 seconds off between sets.

Maini Set: Cardio Pyramid. Climb to the peak, then head back down again.

- 1 minute at 85% effort, 50 seconds off
- 1 minute at 85% effort, 40 seconds off
- 1 minute at 85% effort, 30 seconds off
- 1 minute at 85% effort, 20 seconds off
- 1 minute at 85% effort, 10 seconds off—You've reached the peak!
- Now turn around and repeat 20 seconds off, 30, 40, until you're back at 50 seconds off ➤

Cool Down: Go easy for two minutes

Recovery

Diaphragm Smash	Hamstring Smash
4 minutes ➤	2 minutes per leg

MOVEMENT PRACTICE: Circuit One—1x

Founder

2x 15-second holds, 10-second rest between ➤

Hip Hinge

12x ➤

Lunge Stretch + Knee Drop

2x 15-second holds, 10 knee drops, per side

Circuit Two—1x

Wide Founder with Tracing + Hold + Gorilla Reaches

- 7x Traces
- 10-second holds
- 10x Gorilla Reaches alternating arms ➤

Body Weight Squat

12x ➤

Woodpecker

- 15-second holds
- 10 hinges
- 10 rotations, per side

Circuit Three—4x

Pushups

5 explosive, full range reps, 30-second rest between all 4 sets

Core Round—1x

Roll-Outs on Stability Ball

Draw the alphabet A–L ➤

Janda Crunch

7x ➤

Side Plank

3x 10-second hold per side, 10-second rest between

Goblet Squat Hold—2 minutes

Cardio

30 minutes of low-intensity, base-building cardio at 60–70% exertion.

Recovery

Lat-to-Rotator Cuff Roll

2 minutes per side ➤

Pigeon Stretch

2 minutes per side

Activation—1x

Ankle Mobility	Bird Dogs	T-Spine Rotations	Glute Bridges	Goblet Squat	Behind the Back Hinge
10 pulses outward, middle and inward for each ankle ➤	10x alternating sides ➤	10x per side ➤	10x bridges, 10x extensions ➤	10x ➤	10x

Core Round—2x

Roll-Outs on Stability Ball	Janda Crunch
Draw the alphabet A–L ➤	7x

Circuit One—2x

Hinge Row	Bulgarian Split Squat	Goblet Squat Walk
10x ➤	10x per side ➤	30-second walk

Circuit Two—2x

Single-arm Floor Press	Kettlebell Dead Lifts	Getups
10x per side ➤	10x ➤	1x per side

Cardio

Warm Up	Main Set	Cool Down
1 minute easy, 2x 30-seconds at 80% effort, with 30 seconds off between sets ➤	• 5x 1 minute at 85–90% effort, 2 minutes recovery pace between ➤	Go easy for two minutes

Recovery

Pec Smash	Hamstring Smash
2 minutes per pec ➤	2 minutes per sleg

Activation—1x

Ankle Mobility	Bird Dogs	T-Spine Rotations	Glute Bridges	Goblet Squat	Behind the Back Hinge
10 pulses outward, middle and inward for each ankle ➤	10x alternating sides ➤	10x per side ➤	10x bridges, 10x extensions ➤	10x ➤	10x

Core Round—2x

Roll-Outs on Stability Ball	Janda Crunch
Draw the alphabet A–Z ➤	7x

Circuit One—3x

Hinge Row	Bulgarian Split Squat	Farmer Carries
8x ➤	8x per side ➤	30-second walk

Circuit Two—3x

Single-arm Floor Press	Kettlebell Dead Lifts	Getups
8x per side ➤	8x ➤	1x per side

Cardio

Warm Up	Main Set	Cool Down
1 minute easy, 2x 30-seconds at 80% effort, with 30 seconds off between sets ➤	• 6x 30 seconds at 90–95% effort, 40 seconds recovery pace between sets ➤	Go easy for two minutes

Recovery

Couch Stretch	T-Spine Smash
2 minutes per side ➤	4 minutes

MOVEMENT PRACTICE: Circuit One—1x

Founder

4x 10-second holds, 10-second rest between ➤

Hip Hinge

12x ➤

Lunge Stretch + Knee Drop

- 2x 10-second hold
- 10 knee drops, per side

Circuit Two—1x

Wide Founder with Tracing + Hold + Gorilla Reaches

- 7x Traces
- 10-second holds
- 10x Gorilla Reaches alternating arms ➤

Body Weight Squat

12x ➤

Woodpecker

- 15-second holds
- 10 hinges
- 10 rotations, per side

Circuit Three—4x

Pushups

5 explosive, full range reps, 30-second rest between all 4 sets

Core Round—1x

Roll-Outs on Stability Ball

Draw the alphabet A–L ➤

Janda Crunch

7x ➤

Side Plank

2x 15-second hold per side, 10-second rest between

Goblet Squat Hold—2 minutes

Cardio

Warm Up

1 minute easy, 2x 30-seconds at 80% effort, with 30 seconds off between sets ➤

Main Set

- 6x 15-second sprints at 95% effort, 1 minute rest between sprints ➤

Cool Down

Go easy for two minutes

Recovery

Glute/TFL Smash

2 minutes per side ➤

Psoas Smash

2 minutes per side

Activation—1x

Ankle Mobility	Bird Dogs	T-Spine Rotations	Glute Bridges	Goblet Squat	Behind the Back Hinge
10 pulses outward, middle and inward for each ankle ➤	10x alternating sides ➤	10x per side ➤	10x bridges, 10x extensions ➤	10x ➤	10x

Core Round—2x

Roll-Outs on Stability Ball	Janda Crunch
Draw the alphabet A–L ➤	7x

Circuit One—3x

Hinge Row	Bulgarian Split Squat	Farmer Carries
8x ➤	8x per side ➤	30-second walk

Circuit Two—3x

Single-arm Floor Press	Kettlebell Dead Lifts	Getups
8x per side ➤	8x ➤	1x per side

Cardio

Time Trial: Challenge yourself and improve your time from Week One. Use the same cardio machine.

Warm Up: 1 minute easy, 2x 30-seconds at 80% effort with 30 seconds off between sets.

- Stationary bike: Pedal 3 miles
- Rower or skier: 2000 meters
- Treadmill: 1.5 miles
- Elliptical: 1.5 miles
- Versa Climber: 1,500 feet

Cool Down: Go easy for two minutes

Recovery

Pec Smash	Hamstring Smash
2 minutes per pec ➤	2 minutes per leg

Circuit One—1x

Founder

3x 15-second holds, 10-second rest between ➤

Hip Hinge

12x ➤

Lunge Stretch + Knee Drop

• 2x 10-second hold
• 10 knee drops, per side

Circuit Two—1x

Wide Founder with Tracing + Hold + Gorilla Reaches

• 7x Traces
• 10-second holds
• 10x Gorilla Reaches alternating arms ➤

Body Weight Squat

12x ➤

Woodpecker

• 15-second holds
• 10 hinges
• 10 rotations, per side

Circuit Three—2x

Pushups

4x 5 explosive, full range reps, 30 second rest in between ➤

Kettlebell Swings

4x 5, 30 second rest in between

Core Round—1x

Roll-Outs on Stability Ball

Draw the alphabet A–Z ➤

Janda Crunch

7x ➤

Side Plank

2x 15-second hold per side, 10-second rest between

Goblet Squat Hold—2 minutes

Cardio

20 minutes of easy, low-intensity cardio at 60–70% exertion.

Recovery

Diaphragm Smash

4 minutes ➤

Hamstring Smash

2 minutes per leg, contract five seconds, release and go deeper into the stretch

Activation—1x

Ankle Mobility	Bird Dogs	T-Spine Rotations	Glute Bridges	Goblet Squat	Behind the Back Hinge
10 pulses outward, middle and inward for each ankle ➤	10x alternating sides ➤	10x per side ➤	10x bridges, 10x extensions ➤	10x ➤	10x

Core Round—1x

Roll-Outs on Stability Ball	Janda Crunch
Draw the alphabet A–Z ➤	7x

Circuit One—2x

Hinge Row	Bulgarian Split Squat	Farmer Carries
8x ➤	8x per side ➤	30-second walk

Circuit Two—2x

Single-arm Floor Press	Kettlebell Dead Lifts	Getups
8x per side ➤	8x ➤	1x per side

Cardio

Warm Up	Main Set: Sprint Series—3x	Cool Down
1 minute easy, 2x 30-seconds at 80% effort, with 30 seconds off between sets ➤	4x 10-second sprints at 90–95% effort, 30 second recovery pace between sprints, 2 minute rest between sets ➤	Go easy for two minutes

Recovery

Lat-to-Rotator Cuff Roll	Pigeon Stretch
2 minutes per side ➤	2 minutes per side

Circuit One—1x

Founder

3x 15-second holds, 10-second rest between ➤

Hip Hinge

12x ➤

Lunge Stretch + Knee Drop

- 2x 10-second hold
- 10 knee drops, per side

Circuit Two—1x

Wide Founder with Tracing + Hold + Gorilla Reaches

- 7x Traces
- 10-second holds
- 10x Gorilla Reaches alternating arms ➤

Body Weight Squat

12x ➤

Woodpecker

- 15-second holds
- 10 hinges
- 10 rotations, per side

Circuit Three—2x

Pushups

4x 5 explosive, full-range reps, 30 seconds rest in between ➤

Kettlebell Swings

4x 5, 30 second rest in between

Core Round—1x

Roll-Outs on Stability Ball

Draw the alphabet A–Z ➤

Janda Crunch

7x ➤

Side Plank

2x 15-second holds, rest 10 seconds between sets, switch sides

Goblet Squat Hold—60 seconds

Cardio

20 minutes of base-building cardio

Recovery

Adductor Stretch

2 minutes per side ➤

Calf Smash

2 minutes per side, rolling slowly over tight spots.

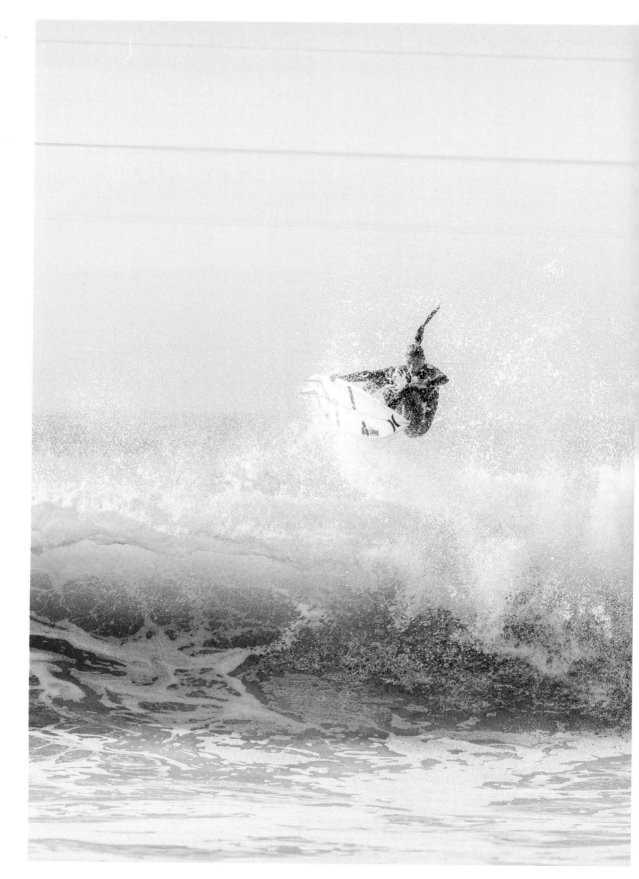

CHAPTER TEN: RINCON

BEFORE MY ULTRA-MARATHON ADDICTION I had a pretty nasty triathlon habit. Before triathlons I was body-building obsessed. Before body building I lived and breathed for the sport of volleyball. And before volleyball, surfing was my everything. Sadly, I don't have time to surf anymore, mostly because three to five days a week I drive the two-hundred-mile roundtrip from Santa Barbara to LA to train clients. My favorite part of the drive back home from the big city is a short span of Highway 101 just inside the Santa Barbara County line that takes me past Rincon Beach where I used to surf as a kid.

Rincon is a rocky, west-facing jut of seashore and one of Southern California's best surfing beaches. When the swell makes it past the Channel Islands, the surf gets good there. These days I experience Rincon vicariously through the surfers I've worked with, like Kelly Slater, Alex Gray, and Lakey Peterson. Have fun with Rincon. For me.

NEW EXERCISES

> SINGLE-LEG ROMANIAN DEAD LIFTS

Why perform a Romanian dead lift with one leg when you can get the exercise done in half the time with two? As with Bulgarian split squats, isolating one leg at a time helps overcome imbalances you might have developed over the years.

Single-leg RDLs are a balancing act and, as such, draw in accessory and stabilizer muscles as you hinge back on one leg. They really isolate the hamstrings, glutes, and posterior chain. Use kettlebells or dumbbells, whichever you prefer.

Start by standing with your feet shoulder-width apart. Lock your lats, pack your shoulders down, and make sure your back is flat. Take in a sniff of air, and brace your abs. Keeping the weights and your own weight positioned over your midfoot, sink into the left hip, and hinge forward as far as you can, keeping your front knee slightly bent, shin vertical, and hips stay square as you're sinking into the hinge. Keep going until you feel a stretch in your hamstrings and glutes. Don't let your body rotate and open, or you'll get out of your hamstring and lose hip stability.

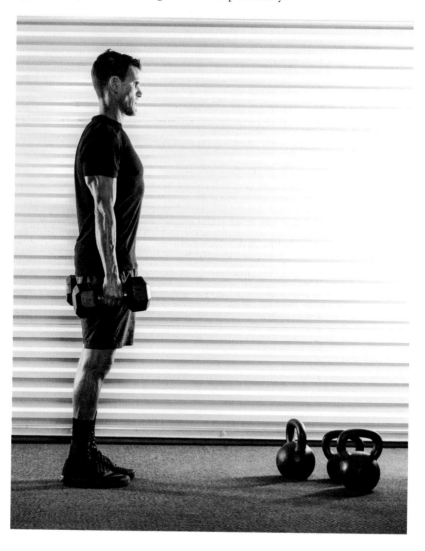

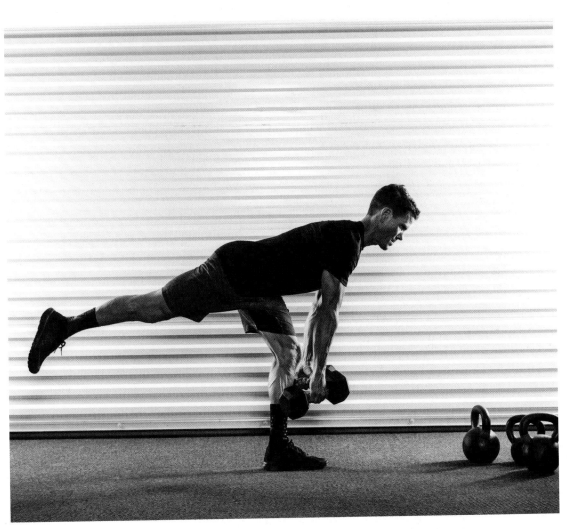

Now, pull with your glute and hamstrings to get back up into the starting position. Rebrace for the next rep. Repeat on opposite leg.

> BENCH PRESS WITH DUMBBELLS

By creating tension in your feet and squeezing your glutes tightly, you engage the lower body and core into the exercise, making it more efficient and powerful.

The safest way to get into the starting position with dumbbells is to take a seat on a bench, the dumbbells resting on your lower quads, just above your knees. Now, roll backward, taking the weights with you. Extend your arms with the weights above you.

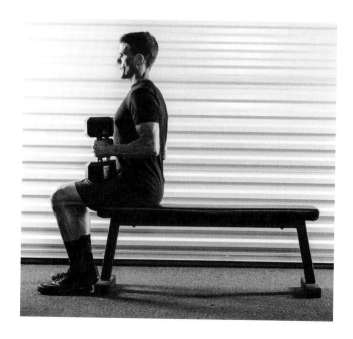

Lying on your back, plant your feet wide and bend your legs to around 90 degrees. Push your feet into the floor to create lower-body tension, then squeeze your glutes. Take a sniff of air, and brace your abs.

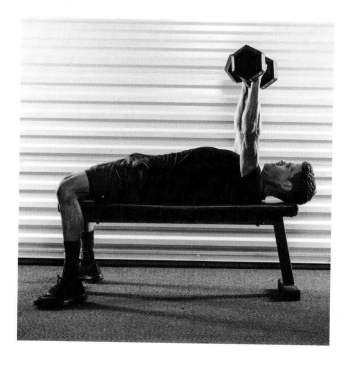

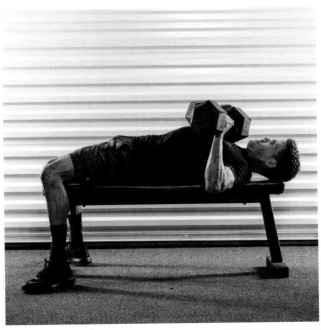

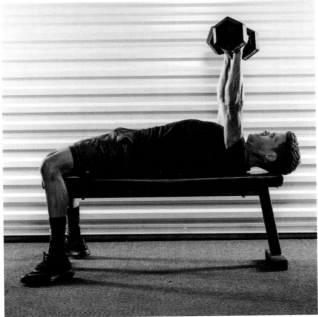

As you row the weights down, be sure to keep your shoulders packed into the bench. Lower the weights until you begin to feel a stretch in your chest. Rebrace your abs, and drive the weights back to the top.

> HINGE ROW WITH FIVE-SECOND HOLD AT THE END POINT

Follow the same exercise cues as the hinge row (page 150), but now squeeze your shoulder blades together, and hold the weights at the end point for five seconds before rowing them down slowly. Rebrace for the next rep.

> SLOW ECCENTRIC GOBLET SQUATS

Taking five seconds to lower yourself to the bottom of your squat increases time under tension, stress to your muscles, and makes the squat more challenging.

Follow the same cues as goblet squat (page 117). Lock your lats, and pack your shoulders down. Take a sniff in, and brace your abs. Slowly, taking five seconds, pull yourself down to the bottom of the squat, keeping your shins as vertical as possible. Rebrace, then using a powerful hip drive, push all the way back up to the starting position.

> EIGHT-POINT PLANK WITH REACH-OUTS

Like bird dogs, eight-point plank with reach-outs are an antirotational exercise. To remind you, antirotational means that when you do the movement you'll purposefully put yourself off balance so your body wants to rotate. The workout happens by fighting that rotation using your abs as stablizers, especially the obliques.

Start by getting into the eight-point plank position (see page 72). Take a sniff of air, and brace your abs as tightly as you can.

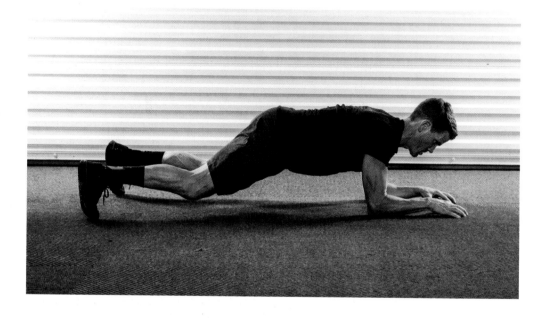

Slowly extend one arm out in front of you, your thumb aiming away from you, and hold it there. Your body shouldn't tilt but remain square to the floor. This is where your obliques kick in to stabilize. Now retract your arm, and get back into eight-point plank, brace again, and extend the other arm.

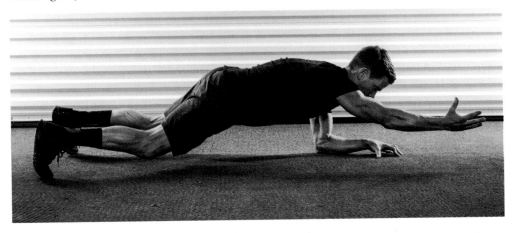

> V-SIT ISOMETRIC CRUNCH

I love this crunch because you're working your whole anterior core, and by squeezing your heels and pushing your hands into the floor, you bring more deep stabilizing muscles into the isometric part of the exercise.

Start on your back with your heels together. Put your hands on the ground next to your hips, with your arms fully extended. Take a sniff of air, brace your abs, and go up into a crunch. Now squeeze your heels and glutes together, and lift your legs six inches off the floor. Push your hands and lower back into the floor to create more tension.

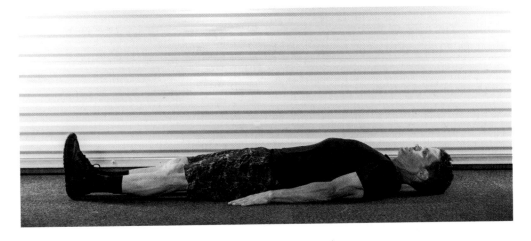

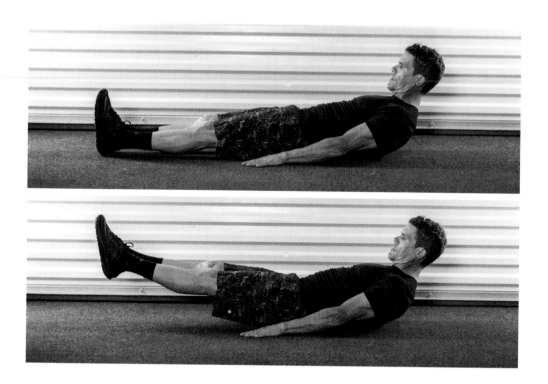

> ONE-ARM FARMER CARRIES

One-arm farmer carries are another antirotational exercise. Remember, as with all carries, perfect posture is key.

Hold a single kettlebell or dumbbell at your side. Pull your shoulders down and back, and don't let the weight tilt you to one side. Now, walk for the prescribed time, focusing on maintaining good posture. You should feel the activation of your core stabilizers on the side opposite the weight. Switch the weight to your other arm and go again.

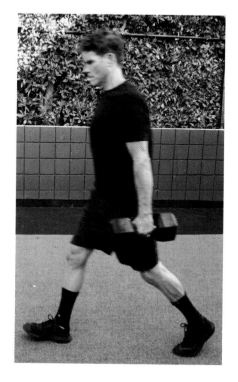

> BULGARIAN SPLIT SQUATS IN GOBLET SQUAT POSITION

The movement of this exercise is identical to Bulgarian split squats, so you already know how to do it. The only difference is that instead of holding weights at your sides, you're going to front load your anterior core. When you're holding the weight at chest-height, make sure you pull your shoulders down and lock your lats, stabilizing your upper back.

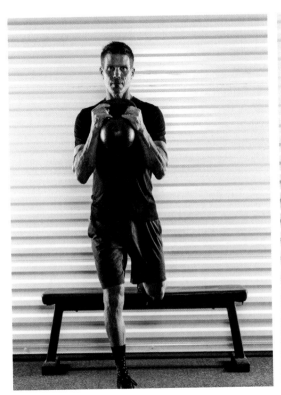 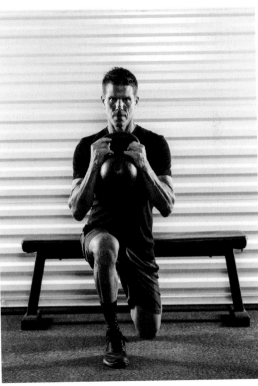

RINCON: WEEK ONE ➤ DAY ONE

Activation—1x

Ankle Mobility	Bird Dogs	T-Spine Rotations	Glute Bridges	Goblet Squat	Behind the Back Hinge
10 pulses outward, middle and inward for each ankle ➤	10x alternating sides ➤	10x per side ➤	10x bridges, 10x extensions ➤	10x ➤	10x

Core Round—2x

V-sit Isometric Crunch	Eight-Point Plank
3x 10-second all-out tension, 10-second rest between ➤	4x 3-second reach-outs, alternating sides

Circuit One—2x

Hinge Row with 5-second Hold	Slow, Eccentric Squat	One-Arm Farmer Carries
5x per side ➤	5x taking 5 seconds to reach bottom of squat, power back to top ➤	30-second walk , per arm

Circuit Two—3x

Dumbbell Bench Press	Single-leg Romanian Dead Lifts
10x ➤	10x per side

Cardio

Warm Up	Main Set	Cool Down
1 minute easy, 2x 30-seconds at 80% effort, with 30 seconds off between sets ➤	2x 5 minutes at 80% effort, 2 minutes recovery pace between sets ➤	Go easy for two minutes

Recovery

Couch Stretch	T-Spine Smash
2 minutes per side ➤	4 minutes

MOVEMENT PRACTICE: Circuit One—1x

Founder

4x 10-second holds, 10-second rest between ➤

Hip Hinge

12x ➤

Lunge Stretch + Knee Drop

2x 10-second holds, 10 knee drops, per side

Circuit Two—1x

Wide Founder with Tracing + Hold + Gorilla Reaches

- 7x Traces
- 10-second holds
- 10x Gorilla Reaches alternating arms ➤

Body Weight Squat

12x ➤

Woodpecker

- 15-second holds
- 10 hinges
- 10 rotations, per side

Circuit Three—2x

Pushups

4x 5 explosive full-range reps, 30-second rest between ➤

Kettlebell Swings

4x 7 with 30-second rest between

Core Round—5x

Getups

1 per side

Goblet Squat Hold—2.5 minutes

Cardio

Warm Up: 1 minute easy, 2x 30-seconds at 80% effort with 30 seconds off between sets.

Main Set: Choose Two Cardio Machines

2x First Machine
- 4x 7-second sprints at 95% effort, 30-second rest between sprints
- 1-minute rest between sets

2x Second Machine
- 4x 7-second sprints at 95% effort, 30-second rest between sprints
- 1-minute rest between sets

Cool Down: Go easy for two minutes

Recovery

Glute/TFL Smash

2 minutes per side ➤

Psoas Smash

2 minutes per side

Activation—1x

Ankle Mobility	Bird Dogs	T-Spine Rotations	Glute Bridges	Goblet Squat	Behind the Back Hinge
10 pulses outward, middle and inward for each ankle ➤	10x alternating sides ➤	10x per side ➤	10x bridges, 10x extensions ➤	10x ➤	10x

Core Round—2x

V-sit Isometric Crunch

3x 10-second all-out tension, 10-second rest between ➤

Eight-Point Plank

4x 3-second reach-outs, alternating sides

Circuit One—2x

Hinge Row with 5-second Hold

5x per side ➤

Slow, Eccentric Squat

5x taking 5 seconds to reach bottom of squat, power back to top ➤

One-Arm Farmer Carries

30-second walk , per arm

Circuit Two—2x

Dumbbell Bench Press

10x ➤

Single-leg Romanian Dead Lifts

10x per side

Cardio

Warm Up

1 minute easy, 2x 30-seconds at 80% effort, with 30 seconds off between sets ➤

Main Set—2x

• 5x 40-second sprints at 80–85% effort, 20 seconds at recovery pace between sprints
• 2 minute rest between the two sets ➤

Cool Down

Go easy for two minutes

Recovery

Pec Smash

2 minutes per pec ➤

Hamstring Smash

2 minutes per leg

Activation—1x

Ankle Mobility	Bird Dogs	T-Spine Rotations	Glute Bridges	Goblet Squat	Behind the Back Hinge
10 pulses outward, middle and inward for each ankle ➤	10x alternating sides ➤	10x per side ➤	10x bridges, 10x extensions ➤	10x ➤	10x

Core Round—2x

V-sit Isometric Crunch	Eight-Point Plank
3x 10-second all-out tension, 10-second rest between ➤	4x 5-second reach-outs, alternating sides

Circuit One—2x

Bench Row	Bulgarian Split Squat, Weight in Goblet Position	One-Arm Farmer Carries
10x per side ➤	10x per leg ➤	30-second walk , per arm, be mindful of your posture, keeping shoulders packed down

Circuit Two—3x

Dumbbell Bench Press	Single-leg Romanian Dead Lifts
10x ➤	10x per side, square your hips as you sink into the hinge

Cardio

Warm Up	Main Set—2x	Cool Down
1 minute easy, 2x 30-seconds at 80% effort, with 30 seconds off between sets ➤	• 8x 20-second sprints at 80–85% effort, 10 second recovery pace between sprints • 3 minutes of low-intensity pace • 6x 10-second sprints at 95% effort, 30 second rest between sprints ➤	Go easy for two minutes

Recovery

Diaphragm Smash	Hamstring Smash
4 minutes ➤	2 minutes per side

MOVEMENT PRACTICE: Circuit One—1x

Founder

2x 15-second holds, 10-second rest between, all-out full-tension ➤

Hip Hinge

12x ➤

Lunge Stretch + Knee Drop

2x 10-second holds, 10 knee drops, per side

Circuit Two—1x

Wide Founder with Tracing + Hold + Gorilla Reaches

- 7x Traces
- 10-second holds
- 10x Gorilla Reaches alternating arms ➤

Body Weight Squat

12x ➤

Woodpecker

- 15-second holds
- 10 hinges
- 10 rotations, per side

Circuit Three—2x

Pushups

4x 5 explosive full-range reps, 30-second rest between ➤

Kettlebell Swings

4x 7 with 30-second rest between

Core Round—5x

Getups

1 per side, keep your eyes on the kettlebell until lunge position

Goblet Squat Hold—2.5 minutes

Cardio

30 minutes of low-intensity, base-building, staying under 80% effort.
Optional: 2 different machines, 5 minutes on each, 3x through

Recovery

Pigeon Stretch

2 minutes per side ➤

Lat-to-Rotator Cuff Roll

2 minutes per side

Activation—1x

Ankle Mobility	Bird Dogs	T-Spine Rotations	Glute Bridges	Goblet Squat	Behind the Back Hinge
10 pulses outward, middle and inward for each ankle ➤	10x alternating sides ➤	10x per side ➤	10x bridges, 10x extensions ➤	10x ➤	10x

Core Round—2x

V-sit Isometric Crunch	Eight-Point Plank
3x 10-second all-out tension, 10-second rest between, focus on pushing your hands into the floor to increase core tension ➤	4x 3-second reach-outs, alternating sides, keep your body square to the floor

Circuit One—2x

Bench Row	Bulgarian Split Squat, Weight in Goblet Position	One-Arm Farmer Carries
10x per side ➤	10x per leg ➤	30-second walk , per arm

Circuit Two—3x

Dumbbell Bench Press	Single-leg Romanian Dead Lifts
10x ➤	10x per side

Cardio

Warm Up	Main Set	Cool Down
1 minute easy, 2x 30-seconds at 80% effort, with 30 seconds off between sets ➤	8x 1-minute at 80–85% effort, 30 seconds at recovery pace between ➤	Go easy for two minutes

Recovery

Adductor Stretch	Calf Smash
2 minutes per side ➤	2 minutes per leg

RINCON: WEEK THREE ➤ DAY ONE

Activation—1x

Ankle Mobility	Bird Dogs	T-Spine Rotations	Glute Bridges	Goblet Squat	Behind the Back Hinge
10 pulses outward, middle and inward for each ankle ➤	10x alternating sides ➤	10x per side ➤	10x bridges, 10x extensions ➤	10x ➤	10x

Core Round—2x

Oblique Rolls	Eight-Point Plank
10x per side ➤	2x 10-second reach-outs, alternating sides

Circuit One—3x

Hinge Row with 5-second Hold	Slow, Eccentric Squat	One-Arm Farmer Carries
5x per side ➤	5x taking 5 seconds to reach bottom of squat, power back to top ➤	30-second walk , per arm

Circuit Two—3x

Dumbbell Bench Press	Single-leg Romanian Dead Lifts
8x ➤	8x per side

Cardio

Warm Up	Main Set	Cool Down
1 minute easy, 2x 30-seconds at 80% effort, with 30 seconds off between sets ➤	• 16-minute tempo pace at 80% effort • Every fourth minute increase effort to 85% effort for 1 minute, then go back to 80% for 3 minutes ➤	Go easy for two minutes

Recovery

Couch Stretch	T-Spine Smash
2 minutes per side ➤	4 minutes

MOVEMENT PRACTICE: Circuit One—1x

Founder

2x 15-second holds, 10-second rest between ➤

Hip Hinge

12x ➤

Lunge Stretch + Knee Drop

2x 10-second holds, 10 knee drops, per side

Circuit Two—1x

Wide Founder with Tracing + Hold + Gorilla Reaches

- 7x Traces
- 10-second holds
- 10x Gorilla Reaches alternating arms ➤

Body Weight Squat

12x ➤

Woodpecker

- 15-second holds
- 10 hinges
- 10 rotations, per side

Circuit Three—2x

Pushups

4x 5 explosive full-range reps, 30-second rest between ➤

Kettlebell Swings

4x 7 with 30-second rest between

Core Round—5x

Getups

1 per side, keep your eyes on the kettlebell until lunge position

> **Goblet Squat Hold—3 minutes, keep your back flat heels on the ground**

Cardio

20 minutes of low-intensity, base-building, staying under 80% effort.
Optional: 3 different machines, 10 minutes on each

Recovery

Glute/TFL Smash

2 minutes per side ➤

Psoas Smash

2 minutes per side

Activation—1x

Ankle Mobility	Bird Dogs	T-Spine Rotations	Glute Bridges	Goblet Squat	Behind the Back Hinge
10 pulses outward, middle and inward for each ankle ➤	10x alternating sides ➤	10x per side ➤	10x bridges, 10x extensions ➤	10x ➤	10x

Core Round—2x

Oblique Rolls	Eight-Point Plank
10x per side ➤	2x 10-second reach-outs, alternating sides

Circuit One—2x

Hinge Row with 5-second Hold	Slow, Eccentric Squat	One-Arm Farmer Carries
5x, rebrace your core before each rep ➤	5x ➤	30-second walk , per arm

Circuit Two—2x

Dumbbell Bench Press	Single-leg Romanian Dead Lifts
8x ➤	8x per side

Cardio

Warm Up: 1 minute easy, 2x 30-seconds at 80% effort with 30 seconds off between sets.

Main Set: 3x on two different cardio machines

- **Machine 1:** 4x 7-second sprints at 95% effort, 30 seconds at recovery pace between sprints
- **Machine 2:** 4x 7-second sprints at 95% effort, 30 seconds at recovery pace between sprints
- Rest one minute between all three rounds

Cool Down: Go easy for two minutes

Recovery

Pec Smash	Hamstring Smash
2 minutes per pec ➤	2 minutes per leg

Circuit One—1x

Founder

3x 15-second holds, 10-second rest between ➤

Body Weight Squat

12x ➤

Woodpecker

- 15-second holds
- 10 hinges
- 10 rotations, per side

Circuit Two—1x

Wide Founder with Tracing + Hold + Gorilla Reaches

- 7x Traces
- 10-second holds
- 10x Gorilla Reaches alternating arms ➤

Lunge Stretch + Knee Drop

2x 10-second holds, then 7x knee drops, per side ➤

Hip Hinges + Tension Hold

12x Hinges, on last one, hold sphere of tension for 15 seconds

Circuit Three—2x

Pushups

4x 5 explosive full-range reps, 30-second rest between ➤

Kettlebell Swings

4x 5, 30-second rest between

Core Round—1x

Roll-outs on Stability Ball

Draw the alphabet A–Z ➤

Janda Crunch

7x ➤

Side Plank

2x 15-second holds, per side, 10-second rest between

Goblet Squat Hold—3 minutes

Cardio

Cross train: 10 minutes of easy, low-intensity cardio at 60–70% exertion on 3 different machines

Recovery

Diaphragm Smash

4 minutes ➤

Hamstring Stretch

2 minutes per side

STRENGTH MAINTENANCE: Activation—1x

Ankle Mobility	Bird Dogs	T-Spine Rotations	Glute Bridges	Goblet Squat	Behind the Back Hinge
10 pulses outward, middle and inward for each ankle ➤	10x alternating sides ➤	10x per side ➤	10x bridges, 10x extensions ➤	10x ➤	10x

Core Round—1x

V-sit Isometric Crunches	Oblique Rolls	Eight-Point Plank
3x 10 seconds, 10 second rest between ➤	10x per side ➤	2x 10-second reach-outs, alternating sides

Circuit One—2x

Hinge Row with 5-second Hold	Slow, Eccentric Squat	Farmer Carries
5x per side ➤	5x taking 5 seconds to reach bottom of squat ➤	30-second walk

Circuit Two—2x

Dumbbell Bench Press	Single-leg Romanian Dead Lifts
8x ➤	8x per side

Cardio

Warm Up: 1 minute easy, 2x 30-seconds at 80% effort with 30 seconds off between sets.

Main Set: Sprint Series—3x

• 4x 10-second sprints at 90–95% effort, 30 seconds recovery pace between sprints
• 2-minute rest sets between sets

Cool Down: Go easy for two minutes

Recovery

Lat-to-Rotator Cuff Roll	Pigeon Stretch
2 minutes per side ➤	2 minutes per side

Circuit One—1x

Founder

3x 15-second holds, 10-second rest between ➤

Body Weight Squat

12x ➤

Woodpecker

- 15-second holds
- 10 hinges
- 10 rotations, per side

Circuit Two—1x

Wide Founder with Tracing + Hold + Gorilla Reaches

- 7x Traces
- 10-second holds
- 10x Gorilla Reaches alternating arms ➤

Lunge Stretch + Knee Drop

2x 10-second holds, then 7x knee drops, per side ➤

Hip Hinge

12x

Circuit Three—2x

Pushups

4x 5 explosive full-range reps, 30-second rest between ➤

Kettlebell Swings

4x 7 with 30-second rest between

Core Round—1x

Roll-outs on Stability Ball

Draw the alphabet A–Z ➤

Janda Crunch

7x ➤

Side Plank

2x 15-second holds, per side, 10-second rest between, sets, switch sides

Goblet Squat Hold—3 minutes

Cardio

30 minutes of low-intensity cross-training on three machines. Use each machine 3x for 5 minutes

Recovery

Adductor Stretch

2 minutes per side ➤

Calf Smash

2 minutes per side, rolling slowly over tight spots

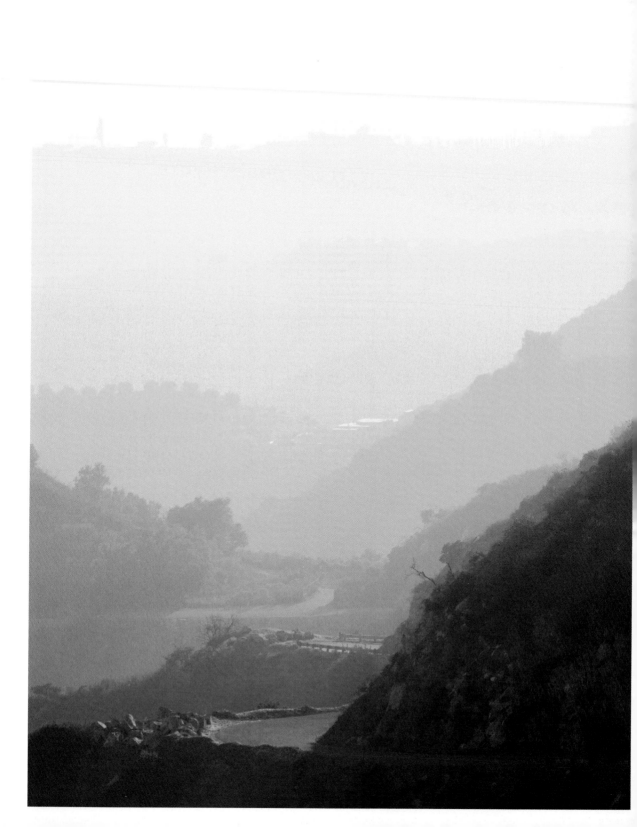

CHAPTER ELEVEN: *GIBRALTAR*

FOR MANY YEARS I DID ONE OF THE TOUGHEST half-marathons you'll ever run, right here in Santa Barbara, known as Pier-to-Peak. It begins at sea level (for about two seconds) and then relentlessly climbs uphill—for four thousand feet. The steepest part of the race is a twisty, windy climb up the road named Gibraltar. In the 2002 race there was an elite out-of-town runner who I knew could give me some trouble. In fact, on any flat course he would've dusted me. But thanks to years of strength training, I'm pretty good on the hills. Plus, I had home-court advantage: I know every nook and cranny of Gibraltar from years of running and biking up it.

When I was about halfway up Gibraltar I was still a minute behind this guy, but I thought he might be going too hard, so I gambled and held my position and waited. I saw my opening as we approached the section of Gibraltar called Flores Flats, where the road flattens out before going into the steepest part of the climb (3 to 4 percent greater than the rest). And sure enough I caught him a half-mile from the top of Gibraltar, passed him, and went on to win the race.

In this workout you're going to do some climbing yourself as you learn two new exercises. The first is pull-overs which will work your lats and help improve shoulder mobility. The second new exercise is a complex—a one-two punch—of Romanian dead lifts followed immediately by lat rows. You're also going to do a new interval training workout called "ins and outs," which keeps your heart rate at its threshold for the duration of the workout. Enjoy Gibraltar.

NEW EXERCISES

> PULL-OVERS

Pull-overs work the lats the same as pull-downs or pull-ups, but they also get your glutes and abs involved and increase your shoulder mobility—a full-body exercise performed on a bench in a bridged position. If you have shoulder issues, and can't do pull-ups, you might still be able to do pull-overs. Give them a try.

Start by sitting on a bench with a dumbbell on your lap. As you lie down on your back, take the dumbbell with you, and raise it above you, with your arms extended and your shoulders packed down. Dig your feet into the bench, take a sniff of air, and brace your abs.

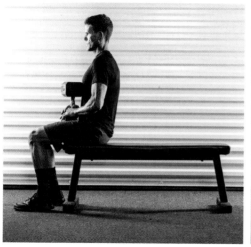 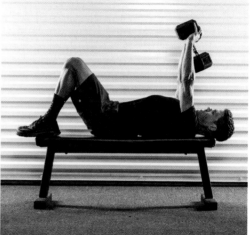

Bridge up, lifting your hips, bracing your core, and squeezing your glutes. Reach back behind you with the weight, keeping your arms straight until you feel a stretch in your lats and shoulders. Make sure your shoulders stay packed down—no shrugging.

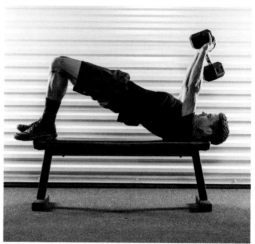

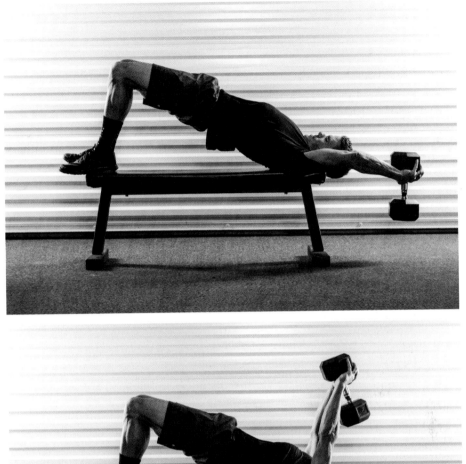

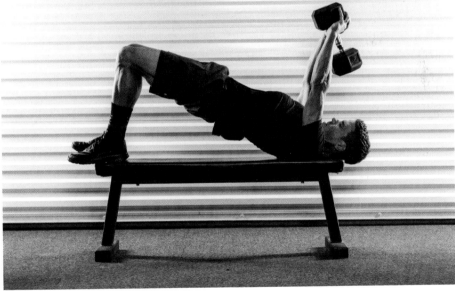

While focusing on using your lats, bring the weight back up with straight arms until you're holding it directly over your face. Rebrace for the next rep. Perform the rest of the reps with your back and hips up in the bridge position.

> ROMANIAN DEAD LIFTS WITH ROWS

You've done RDLs and hip hinge rows. Now we're putting the two together into one dynamic exercise. It's an excellent way to work your entire posterior chain.

Start with your feet shoulder-width apart, holding two weights (kettlebells or dumbbells) at your sides. Corkscrew your feet, squeeze your glutes, take in a sniff of air, and brace your abs.

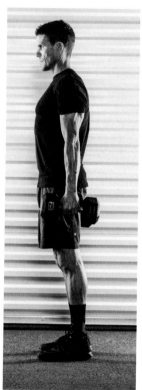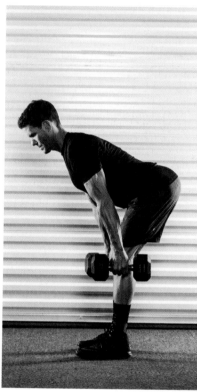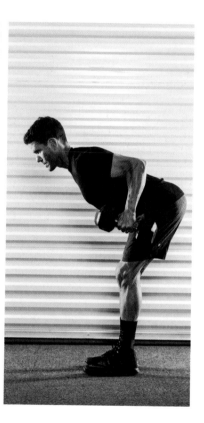

After you do your last dead lift, hold the bottom position, and row the weights up, until your arms reach 90 degrees. Row them slowly back down, rebrace, and then row up again.

> INCLINE BENCH PRESS

I like incline bench press because it isolates the upper chest and shoulders more than a regular bench press.

Start with dumbbells resting on your lower quads.

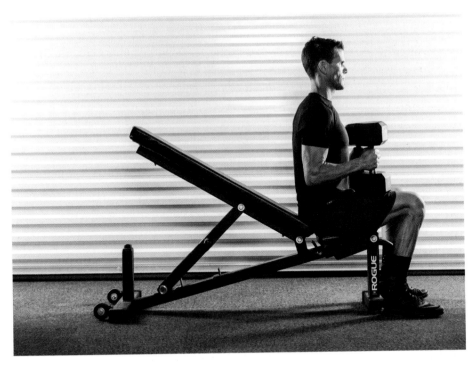

As you lean back, kick the weights up with you, and raise them straight above you.

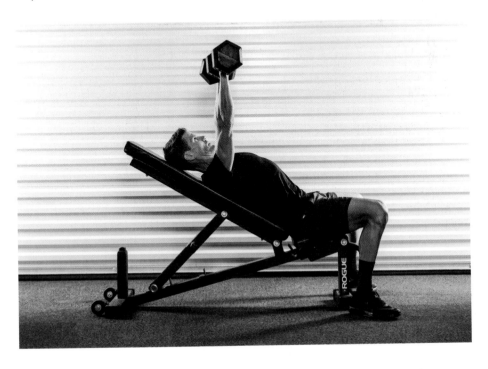

Keeping your shoulders packed down and into the bench, with control, slowly lower the weights down until you feel a stretch. Pause momentarily.

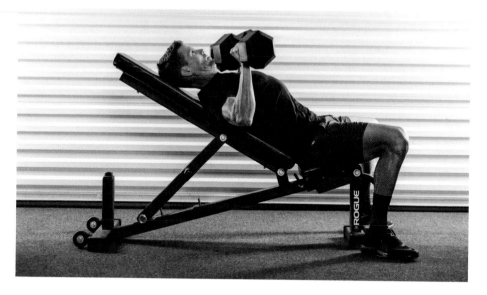

Press the weights back up above you, making sure your shoulders stay back. Re-brace for the next rep.

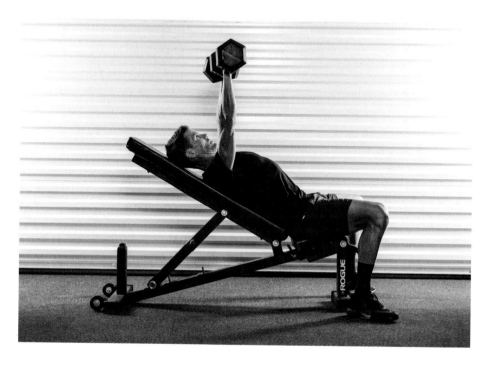

> ONE-ARM INCLINE PRESS

Pressing one arm at a time, an antirotational exercise, forces you to engage your core during the movement to maintain stability.

Lift a medium-weight dumbbell onto your lower quad. Lean back onto the incline bench, and use your knees to push the weight up to the starting position (resting just at your shoulders).

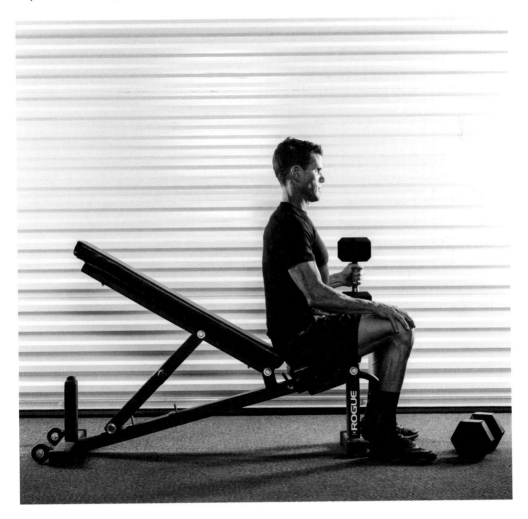

Put your free hand behind your head. Grab the floor with your feet, squeeze your glutes, pack down your shoulders, take in a sniff of air, and brace your abs.

With your wrist locked straight, press the weight above you until your arm is locked. Slowly lower the weight, rebrace for the next rep, and repeat.

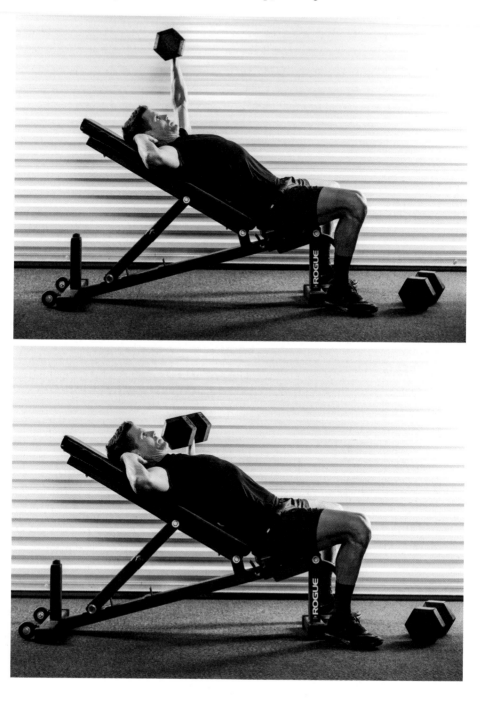

> STANDING PLANK WITH RESISTANCE BAND

This exercise is another antirotational that works the core in a standing upright position. Using the band challenges the core to stay locked in and stable during dynamic motion: your body wants to rotate, but by locking you fight back and challenge the core to stay stable.

Anchor a band on something stable like a squat rack, post, or heavy exercise equipment. Choose a band that's medium tension at first, and increase tension as you get stronger. Take the band with both hands. Walk out (away from the anchor) laterally until you feel the band tense. Lock your arms. Corkscrew your feet into the floor, lock your abs, pull your ribs down, and squeeze your butt. Hold the band out while maintaining the plank, and bring your arms up to slightly above your head and then back down.

For the second part of the exercise, extend your arms fully and draw clockwise circles first, then reverse and go counter-clockwise, maintaining tension the whole time. When you're finished, repeat on the other side.

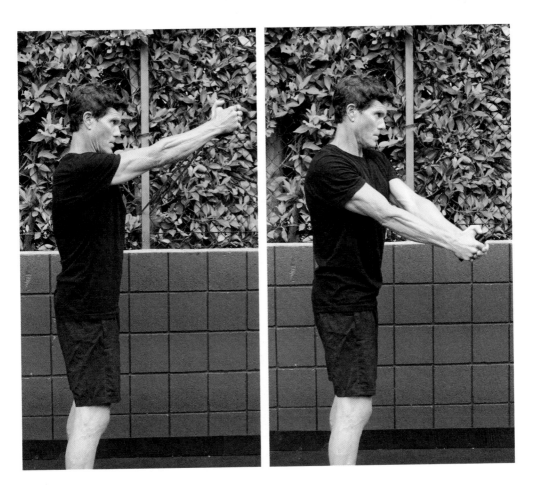

Activation—1x

Ankle Mobility	Bird Dogs	T-Spine Rotations	Glute Bridges	Goblet Squat	Behind the Back Hinge
10 pulses outward, middle and inward for each ankle ➤	10x alternating sides ➤	10x per side ➤	10x bridges, 10x extensions ➤	10x ➤	10x

Core Round—2x

Side Plank	Standing Plank with Band
3x 10-second hold with weight on hip, per side, 10-seconds rest between holds ➤	5x extending straight up and 5x circles, per side

Circuit One—2x

Incline Bench Press	Romanian Dead Lift-into Hip Hinge Rows	Farmer Carries
10x ➤	7x each exercise, no rest between ➤	30-second walk

Circuit Two—2x

Slow, Eccentric Bulgarian Split Squats	Pull-overs	Getups
5x per side ➤	10x ➤	1x per side

Cardio

Warm Up: 1 minute easy, 2x 30-seconds at 80% effort with 30 seconds off between sets.

Main Set: Ins and Outs—6x

2x First Machine
- 1 minute at 80–85% effort
- 1 minute at 70–75% effort

Cool Down: Go easy for two minutes

Recovery

Couch Stretch	T-Spine Smash
2 minutes per side ➤	4 minutes

MOVEMENT PRACTICE: Circuit One—1x

Founder

3x 15-second holds, 10-second rest between ➤

Body Weight Squat

12x ➤

Woodpecker

- 15-second holds
- 10 hinges
- 10 rotations, per side

Circuit Two—1x

Wide Founder with Tracing + Hold + Gorilla Reaches

- 7x Traces
- 10-second holds
- 10x Gorilla Reaches alternating arms ➤

Lunge Stretch + Knee Drop

2x 10-second holds, 10 knee drops, per side ➤

Hip Hinge

12x

Circuit Three—2x

Pushups

4x 5 explosive full-range reps, 30-second rest between ➤

Kettlebell Swings

4x 7 with 30-second rest between

Core Round—5x

Getups

1x per side. Keep your eyes on the kettlebell until lunge position

Goblet Squat Hold—3 minutes

Cardio

15 minutes of low-intensity cardio

Recovery

Pec Smash

2 minutes per pec ➤

Hamstring Smash

2 minutes per leg

Activation—1x

Ankle Mobility	Bird Dogs	T-Spine Rotations	Glute Bridges	Goblet Squat	Behind the Back Hinge
10 pulses outward, middle and inward for each ankle ➤	10x alternating sides ➤	10x per side ➤	10x bridges, 10x extensions ➤	10x ➤	10x

Core Round—2x

Side Plank	Standing Plank with Band
3x 10-second hold with weight on hip, per side, 10-seconds rest between holds ➤	5x extending straight up and 5x circles, per side

Circuit One—2x

Incline Bench Press	Romanian Dead Lift-into Hip Hinge Rows	Farmer Carries
10x ➤	7x each exercise, no rest between ➤	30-second walk

Circuit Two—2x

Slow, Eccentric Bulgarian Split Squats	Pull-overs	Getups
5x per side ➤	10x ➤	1x per side

Cardio

Warm Up: 1 minute easy, 2x 30-seconds at 80% effort with 30 seconds off between sets.

Main Set:

- 4 minutes at 75% effort, 2 minutes easy pace
- 3 minutes at 80% effort, 90 seconds easy pace
- 2 minutes at 85% effort, 1 minute easy pace
- 1 minute at 95% effort

Cool Down: Go easy for two minutes

Recovery

Pec Smash	Hamstring Smash
2 minutes per pec ➤	2 minutes per leg

Activation—1x

Ankle Mobility	Bird Dogs	T-Spine Rotations	Glute Bridges	Goblet Squat	Behind the Back Hinge
10 pulses outward, middle and inward for each ankle ➤	10x alternating sides ➤	10x per side ➤	10x bridges, 10x extensions ➤	10x ➤	10x

Core Round—2x

Janda Crunch	Standing Plank with Band
7x using no momentum to crunch up ➤	7x extending straight up and 7x circles, per side

Circuit One—3x

One-Arm Incline Bench Press	Romanian Dead Lift-into Hip Hinge Rows	Farmer Carries
10x ➤	7x each exercise, no rest between ➤	30-second walk

Circuit Two—2x

Slow, Eccentric Bulgarian Split Squats with 2-second Iso hold at bottom	Pull-overs	Getups
5x per side ➤	10x ➤	1x per side

Cardio

Warm Up: 1 minute easy, 2x 30-seconds at 80% effort with 30 seconds off between sets.

Main Set:

- 2x 2 minutes at 80% effort, 2 minutes rest between
- 2x 1 minute at 85% effort, 1 minute recovery between
- 4x 30-seconds at 90% effort, 30 seconds rest between

Cool Down: Go easy for two minutes

Recovery

Diaphragm Smash	Hamstring Stretch
2 minutes per side ➤	4 minutes

MOVEMENT PRACTICE: Circuit One—1x

Founder

3x 15-second holds, 10-second rest between ➤

Body Weight Squat

12x ➤

Woodpecker

- 15-second holds
- 10 hinges
- 10 rotations, per side

Circuit Two—1x

Wide Founder with Tracing + Hold + Gorilla Reaches

- 7x Traces
- 10-second holds
- 10x Gorilla Reaches alternating arms ➤

Lunge Stretch + Knee Drop

2x 10-second holds, 10 knee drops, per side ➤

Hip Hinge + Tension Hold

12x hinges, on last hinge hold sphere of tension, 20-second

Circuit Three—2x

Pushups

4x 5 explosive full-range reps, 30-second rest between, focus on maintaining perfect form and keeping constant tension ➤

Kettlebell Swings

4x 7 with 30-second rest between, focus on your exploding hip thrust to the top

Core Round—5x

Getups

1x per side

Goblet Squat Hold—3 minutes

Cardio

20 minutes of low-intensity cardio, take it nice and easy

Recovery

Lat-to-Rotator Cuff Roll

2 minutes per side ➤

Pigeon Stretch

2 minutes per leg

Activation—1x

Ankle Mobility	Bird Dogs	T-Spine Rotations	Glute Bridges	Goblet Squat	Behind the Back Hinge
10 pulses outward, middle and inward for each ankle ➤	10x alternating sides ➤	10x per side ➤	10x bridges, 10x extensions ➤	10x ➤	10x

Core Round—2x

Janda Crunch	Standing Plank with Band
7x ➤	7x extending straight up and 7x circles, per side

Circuit One—3x

One-Arm Incline Bench Press	Romanian Dead Lift-into Hip Hinge Rows	Farmer Carries
10x ➤	7x each exercise, no rest between ➤	30-second walk

Circuit Two—3x

Slow, Eccentric Goblet Squats with 2-second Iso hold at bottom	Pull-overs	Getups
5x ➤	10x ➤	1x per side using a more challenging weight

Cardio

Warm Up	Main Set	Cool Down
1 minute easy, 2x 30-seconds at 80% effort, with 30 seconds off between sets ➤	8x 45 seconds at 85% effort, 30 second rest between ➤	Go easy for two minutes

Recovery

Adductor Stretch	Calf Smash
2 minutes per side ➤	2 minutes per leg

Activation—1x

Ankle Mobility	Bird Dogs	T-Spine Rotations	Glute Bridges	Goblet Squat	Behind the Back Hinge
10 pulses outward, middle and inward for each ankle ➤	10x alternating sides ➤	10x per side ➤	10x bridges, 10x extensions ➤	10x ➤	10x

Core Round—2x

Janda Crunch	Weighted Side Plank
7x using no momentum to crunch up ➤	3x 10-second holds, 10 second rest between

Circuit One—3x

Incline Bench Press	Romanian Dead Lift-into Hip Hinge Rows	One-arm Farmer Carries
10x ➤	5x each exercise, no rest between ➤	30-second walk

Circuit Two—2x

Bulgarian Split Squats	Pull-overs	Getups
8x per side ➤	8x ➤	1x per side

Cardio

Warm Up	Main Set	Cool Down
1 minute easy, 2x 30-seconds at 80% effort, with 30 seconds off between sets ➤	2x 6 minutes at 80% effort, 90 second rest between sets ➤	Go easy for two minutes

Recovery

Couch Stretch	T-Spine Smash
2 minutes per side ➤	4 minutes

MOVEMENT PRACTICE: Circuit One—1x

Founder

3x 15-second holds, 10-second rest between ➤

Body Weight Squat

12x ➤

Woodpecker

- 15-second holds
- 10 hinges
- 10 rotations, per side

Circuit Two—1x

Wide Founder with Tracing + Hold + Gorilla Reaches

- 7x Traces
- 10-second holds
- 10x Gorilla Reaches alternating arms ➤

Lunge Stretch + Knee Drop

2x 10-second holds, 10 knee drops, per side ➤

Hip Hinge + Tension Hold

12x hinges, on last hinge hold sphere of tension, 20-seconds

Eight-Point Plank, knees off ground with Reach Outs

2x 5-second holds, alternating sides

Circuit Three—3x

Pushups

2x 10, 45-second rest between, focus on maintaining perfect form and keeping constant tension ➤

Kettlebell Swings

2x 10 with 45-second rest between, focus on your exploding hip thrust to the top

Goblet Squat Hold—3 minutes

Cardio

15 minutes of low-intensity cardio

Recovery

Glute/TFL Smash

2 minutes per side ➤

Psoas Smash

2 minutes per leg

Activation—1x

Ankle Mobility	Bird Dogs	T-Spine Rotations	Glute Bridges	Goblet Squat	Behind the Back Hinge
10 pulses outward, middle and inward for each ankle ➤	10x alternating sides ➤	10x per side ➤	10x bridges, 10x extensions ➤	10x ➤	10x

Core Round—2x

Janda Crunch	Weighted Side Plank
7x ➤	3x 10-second holds, per side

Circuit One—3x

Incline Bench Press	Romanian Dead Lift-into Hip Hinge Rows	One-arm Farmer Carries
8x ➤	8x each exercise, no rest between ➤	30-second walk

Circuit Two—3x

Bulgarian Split Squats	Pull-overs	Getups
8x per side ➤	8x ➤	1x per side using a more challenging weight

Cardio

Warm Up: 1 minute easy, 2x 30-seconds at 80% effort with 30 seconds off between sets.

Main Set: Indoor Triathlon. Choose 3 machines.

- 3x
- 3x 1 minute at 80–85% effort, no rest between
- Rest 2 minutes between

Cool Down: Go easy for two minutes

Recovery

Pec Smash	Hamstring Smash
2 minutes per side ➤	2 minutes per leg

MOVEMENT PRACTICE: Circuit One—1x

Founder

3x 15-second holds, 10-second rest between ➤

Body Weight Squat

12x ➤

Woodpecker

- 15-second holds
- 10 hinges
- 10 rotations, per side

Circuit Two—1x

Wide Founder with Tracing + Hold + Gorilla Reaches

- 7x Traces
- 10-second holds
- 10x Gorilla Reaches alternating arms ➤

Lunge Stretch + Knee Drop

2x 10-second holds, 10 knee drops, per side ➤

Hip Hinge + Tension Hold

12x hinges, on last hinge hold sphere of tension, 20-seconds

Eight-Point Plank, knees off ground with Reach Outs

2x 5-second holds, alternating sides

Circuit Three—3x

Pushups

4x 5 explosive full-range reps, 30-second rest between ➤

Kettlebell Swings

4x 7 with 30-second rest between

Core Round—1x

Roll-outs on Stability Ball

Draw the alphabet A–Z ➤

Janda Crunch

7x ➤

Side Plank

2x 15-second holds, per side, 10-second rest between

> **Goblet Squat Hold—3 minutes**

Cardio

15 minutes of easy, low-intensity cardio at 60–70% exertion.

Recovery

Adductor Stretch

2 minutes per side ➤

Calf Smash

2 minutes per leg, rolling slowly over tight spots.

GIBRALTAR: WEEK FOUR ➤ DAY TWO

STRENGTH MAINTENANCE: Activation—1x

Ankle Mobility	Bird Dogs	T-Spine Rotations	Glute Bridges	Goblet Squat	Behind the Back Hinge
10 pulses outward, middle and inward for each ankle ➤	10x alternating sides ➤	10x per side ➤	10x bridges, 10x extensions ➤	10x ➤	10x

Core Round—2x

Janda Crunch	Standing Plank with Band
7x ➤	10x extending straight up, 10x circles, per side

Circuit One—2x

Incline Bench Press	Romanian Dead Lift-into Hip Hinge Rows	One-arm Farmer Carries
8x ➤	8x each exercise ➤	30-second walk

Circuit Three—2x

Bulgarian Split Squats	Pull-overs
8x per side ➤	8x

Cardio

Warm Up: 1 minute easy, 2x 30-seconds at 80% effort with 30 seconds off between sets.

Main Set: Sprint Series—3x

• 4x 10-second sprints at 95% effort, 30 second recovery between sprints
• 2-minute rest sets between sets

Cool Down: Go easy for two minutes

Recovery

Couch Stretch	T-Spine Smash
2 minutes per side ➤	4 minutes

STRENGTH MAINTENANCE: Activation—1x

Ankle Mobility	Bird Dogs	T-Spine Rotations	Glute Bridges	Goblet Squat	Behind the Back Hinge
10 pulses outward, middle and inward for each ankle ➤	10x alternating sides ➤	10x per side ➤	10x bridges, 10x extensions ➤	10x ➤	10x

Circuit One—5x

Getups

1x per side. Be mindful that you're executing each step of your getup with the best form possible.

Circuit Two—1x

Kettlebell Swings	Pushups
4x 5, 30 second rest in between ➤	4x 5 explosive reps, 30 second rest in between

Goblet Squat Hold—3 minutes

Cardio

30 minutes of low-intensity cross-training on three machines. Use each machine 3x for 5 minutes.

Recovery

Adductor Stretch	Calf Smash
2 minutes per side ➤	2 minutes per leg, rolling slowly over tight spots

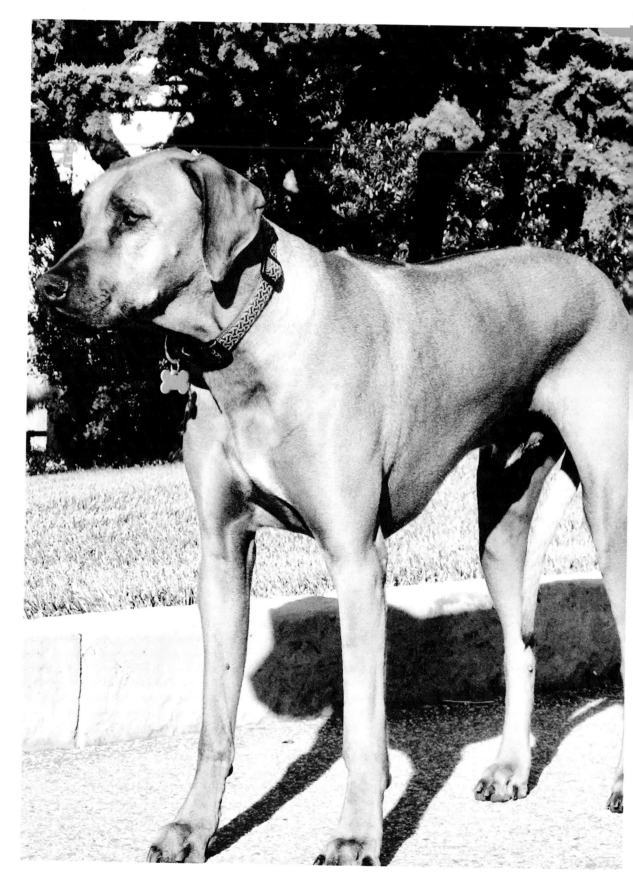

CHAPTER TWELVE: NINE TRAILS

BEFORE I MADE A NAME FOR MYSELF as an athlete, I was known as "the dog guy"—that strange dude who ran Santa Barbara trails with three dogs following behind him. Sadie was my golden retriever, a rescue dog who imprinted so deeply on me that she went to every class I took at UCLA. She wouldn't leave my side. By the time I got my kinesiology degree, she was an expert on human movement too. Sadie trained with me until she grew too old. That nearly broke her heart—and mine too. Clyde was my Anatolian shepherd, a real trooper—what a cool dog he was. But Boomer, my Rhodesian ridgeback, was the dog most like me. No matter how hard I tried, I couldn't wear that dog down. When Boomer was just a year old he ran with me for my first Nine Trails ultra-marathon. The Nine Trails race is only thirty-five miles long, shorter than most ultra-marathons, but the trails are steep, rocky, and practically inaccessible in places, and over the course of those thirty-five miles you climb up ten thousand feet of elevation. Helluva race. Even better when you're in the company of a good dog. Go Boomer!

In Nine Trails you're going to learn two new exercises, single dumbbell hip hinge rows and walking goblet squats. Also, you're going to up your cardio intensity so you can peak for your first time trial. Good luck with Nine Trails.

NEW EXERCISES

> SINGLE-ARM HIP HINGE ROW

Like all single-limb exercise, single-arm hip hinge rows engage the core and focus on developing balance, one side at a time. Use a kettlebell or dumbell.

Begin with your feet shoulder-width apart. Now, get into a hip hinge position while holding a weight in one hand, with your opposite arm fully extended.

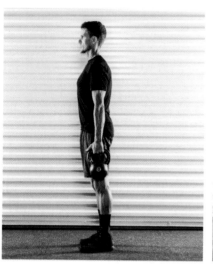 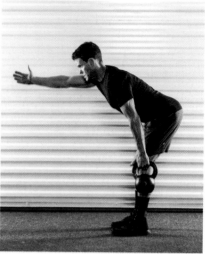

Sniff a breath, brace your abs, then row the weight up, keeping your arm at 90 degrees, and hold for one second before rowing it back down. Make sure your shoulders are packed down and you maintain overall good posture. Rebrace for the next rep.

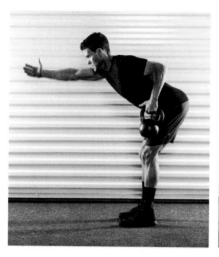 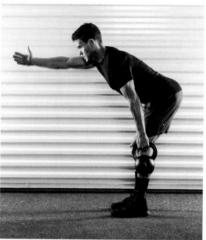

> WALKING GOBLET SQUAT

Squat, walk six steps, squat again, walk another six steps, squat—that's the walking goblet squat. You'll be surprised at how winded this one will get you.

Start with a kettlebell or dumbbell held in goblet position. Create tension, sniff in air, and brace your abs. Do a squat. Now walk five steps, stop, sniff in air, brace, and do another goblet squat. And so on until you've done as many squats as are directed in the workout.

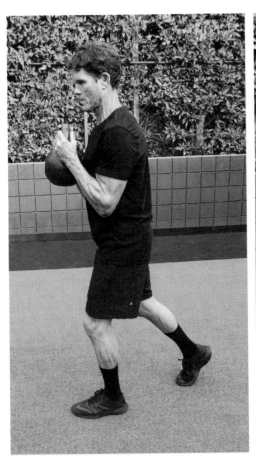 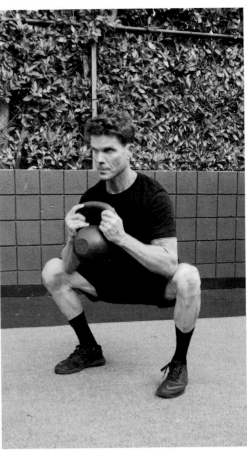

Activation—1x

Ankle Mobility	Bird Dogs	T-Spine Rotations	Glute Bridges	Goblet Squat	Behind the Back Hinge
10 pulses outward, middle and inward for each ankle ➤	10x alternating sides ➤	10x per side ➤	10x bridges, 10x extensions ➤	10x ➤	10x

Core Round—2x

Roll-outs on Stability Ball	V-sit Isometric Crunch
Draw the alphabet A–Z ➤	3x 10-second holds, with 10-second rest between

Circuit One—3x

Single-leg Romanian Dead Lifts	One-Arm Floor Press	Goblet Farmer Carries
10x per side ➤	10x per side ➤	30-second walk

Circuit Two—3x

Walking Goblet Squats	Single-arm Hip Hinge Row	Getups
4x 1 squat, walk 6 steps ➤	10x per side ➤	1x per side

Cardio

Warm Up: 1 minute easy, 2x 30-seconds at 80% effort with 30 seconds off between sets.

Main Set: 2x

- 6x 30-second sprints at 95% effort, 90 second rest between sprints
- Rest 2 minutes between sets 1 and 2

Cool Down: Go easy for two minutes

Recovery

Couch Stretch	T-Spine Smash
2 minutes per side ➤	4 minutes

MOVEMENT PRACTICE: Circuit One—1x

Founder

3x 15-second holds, 10-second rest between ➤

Body Weight Squat

12x ➤

Woodpecker

- 15-second holds
- 10 hinges
- 10 rotations, per side

Circuit Two—1x

Wide Founder with Tracing + Hold + Gorilla Reaches

- 7x Traces
- 10-second holds
- 10x Gorilla Reaches alternating arms ➤

Lunge Stretch + Knee Drop

2x 10-second holds, 7 knee drops, per side

➤

Hip Hinge + Tension Hold

12x hinges, on last hinge hold sphere of tension, 20-seconds

Eight-Point Plank, knees off ground with Reach Outs

1x 10-second holds, per side

Circuit Three—3x

Pushups

2x 10 explosive reps, 45-second rest between ➤

Kettlebell Swings

2x 10 with 45-second rest between

Goblet Squat Hold—3 minutes

Cardio

15 minutes of low-intensity cardio

Recovery

Glute/TFL Smash

2 minutes per side ➤

Psoas Smash

2 minutes per side

Activation—1x

Ankle Mobility	Bird Dogs	T-Spine Rotations	Glute Bridges	Goblet Squat	Behind the Back Hinge
10 pulses outward, middle and inward for each ankle ➤	10x alternating sides ➤	10x per side ➤	10x bridges, 10x extensions ➤	10x ➤	10x

Core Round—2x

Roll-outs on Stability Ball	V-sit Isometric Crunch
Draw the alphabet A–Z ➤	3x 10-second holds, with 10-second rest between

Circuit One—3x

Single-leg Romanian Dead Lifts	One-Arm Floor Press	Farmer Carries
10x per side ➤	10x per side ➤	30-second walk

Circuit Two—3x

Walking Goblet Squats	Single-arm Hip Hinge Row	Getups
4x 1 squat, walk 6 steps ➤	10x per side ➤	1x per side

Cardio

Warm Up	Main Set—4x	Cool Down
1 minute easy, 2x 30-seconds at 80% effort, with 30 seconds off between sets ➤	2-minute intervals at 85% to 90% effort, 1 minute off between intervals ➤	Go easy for two minutes

Recovery

Pec Smash	Hamstring Stretch
2 minutes per side ➤	2 minutes per leg

Activation—1x

Ankle Mobility	Bird Dogs	T-Spine Rotations	Glute Bridges	Goblet Squat	Behind the Back Hinge
10 pulses outward, middle and inward for each ankle ➤	10x alternating sides ➤	10x per side ➤	10x bridges, 10x extensions ➤	10x ➤	10x

Core Round—2x

Oblique Roll

10x per side ➤

Eight-Point Plank

20-second holds, knees off the ground, rest 10 seconds, 2x 5-second alternating Reach-outs

Circuit One—3x

Dead Lifts

10x ➤

Flat Bench Press

10x ➤

One-arm Farmer Carries

30-second walk, per arm

Circuit Two—3x

Slow, Eccentric Bulgarian Split Squats

Take 5 seconds to go down, pause 2 seconds at the bottom, power back to the top ➤

Bench Row

10x per side

Cardio

Warm Up: 1 minute easy, 2x 30-seconds at 80% effort with 30 seconds off between sets.

Main Set: Threshold set. Start conservatively and maintain a threshold pace throughout.
- 6x 90-second sprints at 85–90% effort, 30 second rest between sprints
- Rest 2 minutes between sets 1 and 2

Cool Down: Go easy for two minutes

Recovery

Diaphragm Smash

4 minutes ➤

Hamstring Stretch

2 minutes per leg

MOVEMENT PRACTICE: Circuit One—1x

Founder

3x 20-second holds, 10-second rest between ➤

Body Weight Squat

12x ➤

Woodpecker

- 10-second holds
- 10 hinges
- 10 rotations, per side

Circuit Two—1x

Wide Founder with Tracing + Hold + Gorilla Reaches

- 7x Traces
- 10-second holds
- 10x Gorilla Reaches alternating arms ➤

Lunge Stretch + Knee Drop

2x 10-second holds, 7 knee drops, per side ➤

Hip Hinge + Tension Hold

12x hinges, on last hinge hold sphere of tension, 20-seconds

Eight-Point Plank, knees off ground with Reach Outs

1x 10-second holds, per side

Circuit Three—3x

Pushups

4 to 5 explosive reps, 30-second rest between ➤

Kettlebell Swings

4x 5 with 30-second rest between

Goblet Squat Hold—3 minutes

Cardio

20 minutes of low-intensity cardio

Recovery

Lat-to-Rotator Cuff Roll

2 minutes per side ➤

Pigeon Stretch

2 minutes per side

Activation—1x

Ankle Mobility	Bird Dogs	T-Spine Rotations	Glute Bridges	Goblet Squat	Behind the Back Hinge
10 pulses outward, middle and inward for each ankle ➤	10x alternating sides ➤	10x per side ➤	10x bridges, 10x extensions ➤	10x ➤	10x

Core Round—2x

Oblique Roll	Eight-Point Plank
10x per side ➤	20-second holds, knees off the ground, rest 10 seconds, 2x 5-second alternating Reach-outs, knees on the ground

Circuit One—3x

Dead Lifts	Flat Bench Press	Farmer Carries
10x ➤	10x ➤	30-second walk

Circuit Two—3x

Slow, Eccentric Bulgarian Split Squats	Bench Row
Take 5 seconds to go down, pause 2 seconds at the bottom, power back to the top ➤	10x per side

Cardio

Warm Up: 1 minute easy, 2x 30-seconds at 80% effort with 30 seconds off between sets.

Main Set:
- 4x 15-second intervals at 95–100% effort, 1 minute off between intervals
- 2 minutes recovery
- 4x 15-second intervals at 95–100% effort, 1 minute off between intervals

Cool Down: Go easy for two minutes

Recovery

Pec Smash	Hamstring Smash
2 minutes per side ➤	2 minutes per leg

Activation—1x

Ankle Mobility	Bird Dogs	T-Spine Rotations	Glute Bridges	Goblet Squat	Behind the Back Hinge
10 pulses outward, middle and inward for each ankle ➤	10x alternating sides ➤	10x per side ➤	10x bridges, 10x extensions ➤	10x ➤	10x

Core Round—2x

Roll-outs on Stability Ball	Janda Crunch
Draw the alphabet A–Z ➤	7x

Circuit One—3x

Single-leg Romanian Dead Lifts	Single-Arm Incline Bench Press	One-Arm Farmer Carries
8x ➤	8x per side ➤	30-second walk, per arm

Circuit Two—3x

Walking Goblet Squats	Pull-overs	Getups
4x 2x squat, walk 6 steps ➤	10x per side ➤	1x per side

Cardio

Warm Up: 1 minute easy, 2x 30-seconds at 80% effort with 30 seconds off between sets.

Main Set:

• 5x 20-second sprints at 90–95% effort, 40 seconds off between sprints
• Rest 2 minutes
• 5x 20-second sprints at 95% effort, 45 seconds off between sprints

Cool Down: Go easy for two minutes

Recovery

Couch Stretch	T-Spine Smash
2 minutes per side ➤	4 minutes

MOVEMENT PRACTICE: Circuit One—1x

Founder

3x 15-second holds, 10-second rest between ➤

Body Weight Squat

12x ➤

Woodpecker

- 10-second holds
- 10 hinges
- 10 rotations, per side

Circuit Two—1x

Wide Founder with Tracing + Hold + Gorilla Reaches

- 7x Traces
- 10-second holds
- 10x Gorilla Reaches alternating arms ➤

Lunge Stretch + Knee Drop

2x 10-second holds, 7 knee drops, per side ➤

Hip Hinge + Tension Hold

12x hinges, on last hinge hold sphere of tension, 20-seconds

Eight-Point Plank, knees off ground with Reach Outs

1x 10-second holds, per side

Circuit Three—3x

Pushups

4x 5 explosive reps, 30 second rest between ➤

Kettlebell Swings

4x 7 with 30-second rest between

Goblet Squat Hold—3 minutes

Cardio

Warm Up: 1 minute easy, 2x 30-seconds at 80% effort with 30 seconds off between sets.

Main Set:
- 5x 7-second sprints at 90% effort, 30 seconds off between sprints
- Rest 90 seconds
- 5x 7-second sprints at 95% effort, 30 seconds off between sprints

Cool Down: Go easy for two minutes

Recovery

Glute/TFL Smash

2 minutes per side ➤

Psoas Smash

2 minutes per side

Activation—1x

Ankle Mobility	Bird Dogs	T-Spine Rotations	Glute Bridges	Goblet Squat	Behind the Back Hinge
10 pulses outward, middle and inward for each ankle ➤	10x alternating sides ➤	10x per side ➤	10x bridges, 10x extensions ➤	10x ➤	10x

Core Round—2x

Roll-outs on Stability Ball	Janda Crunch
Draw the alphabet A–Z ➤	7x

Circuit One—3x

Single-leg Romanian Dead Lifts	Single-Arm Incline Bench Press	Farmer Carries
8x per side ➤	8x per side ➤	30-second walk

Circuit Two—3x

Walking Goblet Squats	Pull-overs	Getups
4x	8x ➤	1x
2x squat, walk 6 steps ➤		

Cardio

Warm Up: 1 minute easy, 2x 30-seconds at 80% effort with 30 seconds off between sets.

Main Set: Time Trial. Choose one of the following cardio machines and try to beat your previous time.
- **Stationary bike:** Pedal 3 miles
- **Rower or skier:** 2000 meters
- **Treadmill:** 1.5 miles
- **Elliptical:** 1.5 miles

Cool Down: Go easy for two minutes

Recovery

Pec Smash	Hamstring Smash
2 minutes per side ➤	2 minutes per leg

Circuit One—1x

Founder

3x 15-second holds, 10-second rest between ➤

Body Weight Squat

12x ➤

Woodpecker

- 10-second holds
- 10 hinges
- 10 rotations, per side

Circuit Two—1x

Wide Founder with Tracing + Hold + Gorilla Reaches

- 7x Traces
- 10-second holds
- 10x Gorilla Reaches alternating arms ➤

Lunge Stretch + Knee Drop

2x 10-second holds, 10 knee drops, per side

➤

Hip Hinge + Tension Hold

12x hinges, on last hinge hold sphere of tension, 20-seconds

Eight-Point Plank, knees off ground with Reach Outs

2x 5-second holds, alternating sides

Goblet Squat Hold—3 minutes

Cardio

30 minutes of easy, low-intensity cardio at 60–70% exertion.

Recovery

Hamstring Smash

2 minutes per side ➤

Diaphragm Smash

4 minutes

STRENGTH MAINTENANCE: Activation—1x

Ankle Mobility	Bird Dogs	T-Spine Rotations	Glute Bridges	Goblet Squat	Behind the Back Hinge
10 pulses outward, middle and inward for each ankle ➤	10x alternating sides ➤	10x per side ➤	10x bridges, 10x extensions ➤	10x ➤	10x

Core Round—1x

Getups
5x per side

Circuit One—2x

Kettlebell Dead Lifts	Flat Bench Press	One-Arm Farmer Carries
8x per side ➤	8x ➤	30-second walk, per arm

Circuit Two—2x

Bulgarian Split Squats	Bench Rows
8x per side ➤	8x per side

Cardio

Warm Up: 1 minute easy, 2x 30-seconds at 80% effort with 30 seconds off between sets.

Main Set: Sprint Series—3x

- 4x 10-second sprints at 95% effort, 30 second recovery between sprints
- 2-minute rest sets between sets

Cool Down: Go easy for two minutes

Recovery

Lat-to-Rotator Cuff Roll	Pigeon Stretch
2 minutes per side ➤	2 minutes per side

Circuit One—1x

Founder

3x 15-second holds, 10-second rest between ➤

Body Weight Squat

12x ➤

Woodpecker

- 10-second holds
- 10 hinges
- 10 rotations, per side

Circuit Two—1x

Wide Founder with Tracing + Hold + Gorilla Reaches

- 7x Traces
- 10-second holds
- 10x Gorilla Reaches alternating arms ➤

Lunge Stretch + Knee Drop

2x 10-second holds, 10 knee drops, per side ➤

Hip Hinge + Tension Hold

12x hinges, on last hinge hold sphere of tension, 20-seconds

Eight-Point Plank, knees off ground with Reach Outs

2x 5-second holds, alternating sides

Circuit Three—3x

Kettlebell Swings

2x 10 reps, 45-second rest in between ➤

Pushups

2x 10 explosive reps, 45-second rest in between

Goblet Squat Hold—3 minutes

Cardio

20 minutes of low-intensity cardio

Recovery

Adductor Stretch

2 minutes per side ➤

Calf Smash

2 minutes per side, rolling slowly over tight spots

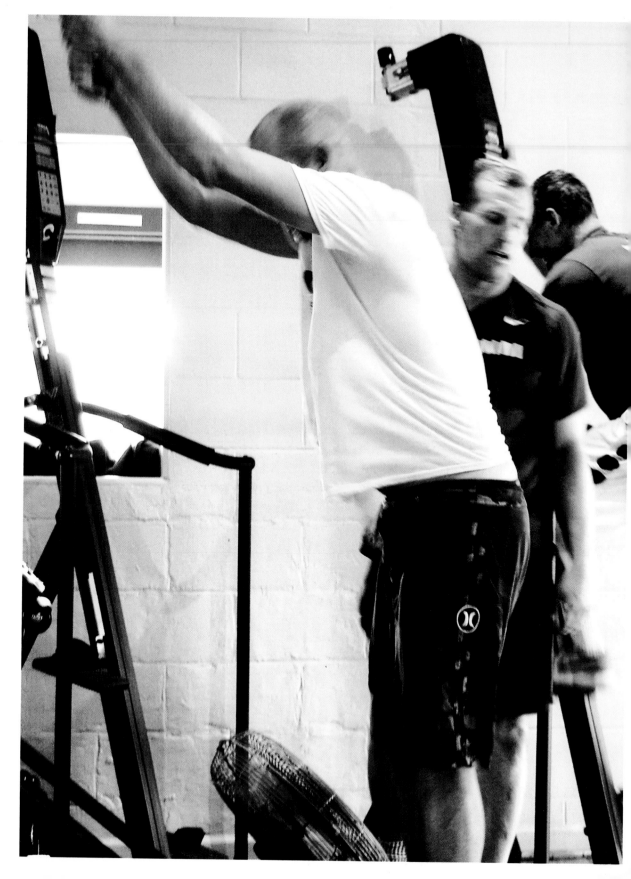

CHAPTER THIRTEEN: SATURDAY MORNINGS

EVERY SATURDAY MORNING John, Chip, Mike, and regulars Steve Shlens, Ryan Leeton, and when she's not off competing, pro surfer Lakey Peterson, join me for a grind-out that combines strength circuits and cardio—a twofer that builds next-level fitness.

These workouts are a true challenge, and not one you have to accept. You could go back and revisit East Beach, Gibraltar, Rincon, or Romero Canyon and make your way through all the workouts again. If you choose to go that route, add more weight, do extra circuits (go for three sets where I ask for two), and concentrate even more intently on creating that tension and utilizing your whole body in each workout. Or join me and the other guys for the Saturday Mornings challenge.

The Saturday Mornings exercise set is structured a bit differently from the other workouts. You'll note that Day One and Day Three will be different workouts. Also, you're going to do fewer reps, move faster, and execute the exercises with explosiveness. Why? To build true power. Make sure you don't go to failure, however, and that the weight you use is light enough that you can maintain perfect technique.

NEW EXERCISES

> EIGHT-POINT PLANK ROW AND EIGHT-POINT PLANK ROW WITH HOLDS

By now you already intimately know the eight-point plank. Now it's time to hook up with its more interesting and challenging cousin, the eight-point plank row. The eight-point plank row is an antirotational exercise that forces you to stabilize your core in order to row a weight up one arm at a time while keeping your body square with the floor. It ain't easy! Rows are primarily a lat-back exercise, but again, by using tension and drawing the core into the movement for stability, you're teaching many parts of your body to work together.

Start in Bird Dog position with two lightweight dumbbells on the floor in front of you. Grab the dumbbells, making sure they're directly underneath your shoulders. Make sure your back is flat, your shoulders are packed, and your lats are locked. Now, bring your knees one to two inches off the ground. Take a sniff of air, and brace your core.

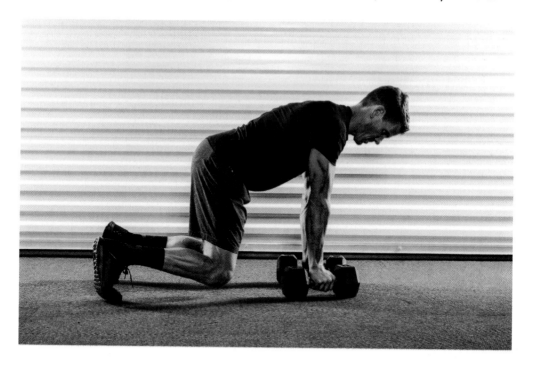

Slowly row one dumbbell up, keeping your shoulders packed and your body stiff and square to the floor. Now slowly return the dumbbell, with control, to the floor. Rebrace your core, and row the other side.

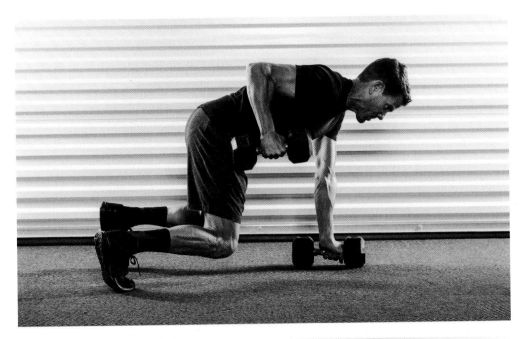

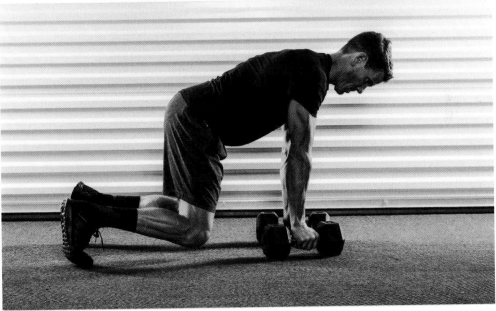

To do the eight-point-plank row with holds, row the weight up, then hold it for a two-count before putting it back to the floor. Two seconds doesn't sound long, but it might prove tougher than you think.

> PUSHUP WALK

Pushup walks are exactly that: do a pushup, then, while at the top of plank position, walk one step laterally with your hands and feet, and then do another. And another. And another, and then make your way back to where you started. What makes Pushup Walks different from normal pushups? Moving laterally engages your core and requires a lot of stability, so you're working a lot of stabilizing muscles as well.

The keys to doing a proper pushup walk are focusing on executing each rep perfectly, maintaining a braced core, and keeping your back flat.

Start in a plank position, with your heels and knees pushing together and your glutes squeezed tight. Take a sniff of air, and brace your abs. Now do a pushup, then come up, take a lateral step sideways with your hands and feet, get organized, rebrace, and do another pushup.

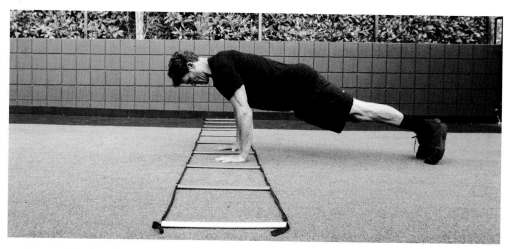

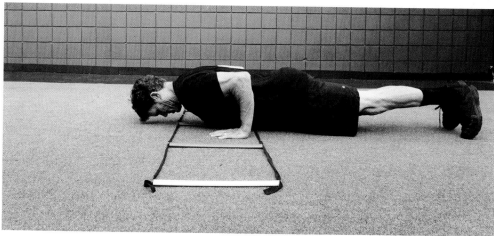

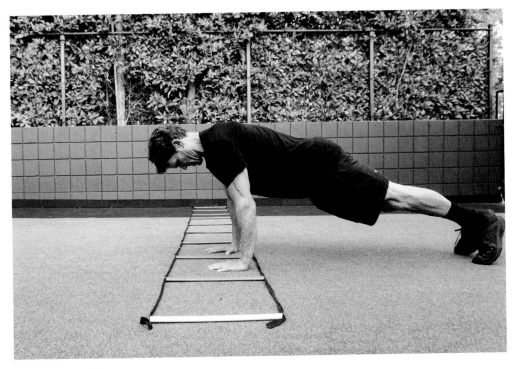

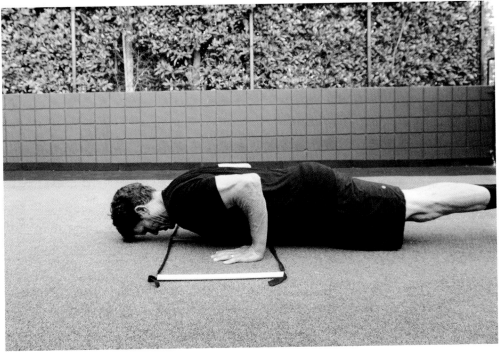

Activation—1x

Ankle Mobility	Bird Dogs	T-Spine Rotations	Glute Bridges	Goblet Squat	Behind the Back Hinge
10 pulses outward, middle and inward for each ankle ➤	10x alternating sides ➤	10x per side ➤	10x bridges, 10x extensions ➤	10x ➤	10x

Core Round—2x

Oblique Rolls	V-sit Isometric Crunch
10x per side ➤	3x 10-second hold all-out tension, 10-second rest between

Circuit One—4x

Bulgarian Split Squats	Pushups	Getup Complex
5x explosive, power up through your glutes and quad ➤	7–10x explosive ➤	5x Punch-Up to Elbow, on the 5th rep do a full Getup, switch sides

Circuit Two—4x

Eight-Point Plank Row	Kettlebell Swing	Farmer Carries
7x per side alternating ➤	10x ➤	30-second walk using challenging weight

Cardio

Warm Up: 1 minute easy, 2x 30-seconds at 80% effort with 30 seconds off between sets.

Main Set: Cross training on two different machines
- **First Machine:** 3x 1 minute on, 1 minute off
- **Second Machine:** 3x 1 minute on, 1 minute off

Cool Down: Go easy for two minutes

Recovery

Couch Stretch	T-Spine Smash
2 minutes per side ➤	4 minutes

Circuit One—1x

Founder

3x 15-second holds, 10-second rest between ➤

Pull-overs

10x ➤

Lunge Stretch + Knee Drop

2x 10-second holds, 7 knee drops, per side

Circuit Two—1x

Wide Founder with Tracing + Hold + Gorilla Reaches

- 7x Traces
- 10-second holds
- 10x Gorilla Reaches alternating arms ➤

Body Weight Squat

12x ➤

Woodpecker

- 15-second holds
- 10 hinges
- 10 rotations, per side

Core Round—1x

Janda Crunch

7x ➤

Weighted Side Plank

3x 10-second holds, per side ➤

Standing Plank with Band

7x extending straight up, 7x circles, per side

Goblet Squat Hold—4.5 minutes

Cardio

30 minutes low-intensity. **Optional:** Go 5 minutes on 3 machines, 2x through.

Recovery

Glute/TFL Smash

2 minutes per pec ➤

Psoas Smash

2 minutes per side

Activation—1x

Ankle Mobility	Bird Dogs	T-Spine Rotations	Glute Bridges	Goblet Squat	Behind the Back Hinge
10 pulses outward, middle and inward for each ankle ➤	10x alternating sides ➤	10x per side ➤	10x bridges, 10x extensions ➤	10x ➤	10x

Core Round—2x

Oblique Rolls	V-sit Isometric Crunch
10x per side ➤	3x 10-second hold all-out tension, 10-second rest between

Circuit One—3x

Goblet Squat Walk	Pushup Walk	Romanian Dead Lift + Hip Hinge Row
4x 2x Goblet Squat, walk 6 steps ➤	Go to 1 before failure ➤	7x per exercise

Circuit Two—3x

Getups	Kettlebell Swing	One-Arm Farmer Carries
1x per side ➤	15x ➤	Walk for 30 seconds, each arm

Cardio

Warm Up: 1 minute easy, 2x 30-seconds at 80% effort with 30 seconds off between sets.

Main Set: Tabata Cardio Workout
- **First Machine:** 8x 20-second sprints at 85–90% effort, 10 second rest
- 2 minutes recovery
- **Second Machine:** 8x 20-second sprints at 85–90% effort, 10 second rest

Cool Down: Go easy for two minutes

Recovery

Pec Smash	Hamstring Smash
2 minutes per side ➤	2 minutes per leg

Activation—1x

Ankle Mobility	Bird Dogs	T-Spine Rotations	Glute Bridges	Goblet Squat	Behind the Back Hinge
10 pulses outward, middle and inward for each ankle ➤	10x alternating sides ➤	10x per side ➤	10x bridges, 10x extensions ➤	10x ➤	10x

Core Round—2x

Standing Plank with Band	Roll-outs on Stability Ball
7x extending straight up, 7x circles, per side ➤	Draw the alphabet A–Z

Circuit One—4x
(30-second maximum rest between each exercise)

Goblet Squat	Flat Bench Press	Getups
5x explosive ➤	5x ➤	1 per side

Circuit Two—4x

Hip Hinge Row	Kettlebell Swing	One-Arm Farmer Carries
10x ➤	12x ➤	30-second walk

Cardio

Warm Up: 1 minute easy, 2x 30-seconds at 80% effort with 30 seconds off between sets.

Main Set: Indoor Triathalon. Choose 3 machines—3x

- 1 minute on each machine, no rest between
- 2 minutes rest between your 3 rounds

Cool Down: Go easy for two minutes

Recovery

Diaphragm Smash	Hamstring Stretch
2 minutes per side ➤	4 minutes

MOVEMENT PRACTICE: Circuit One—1x

Founder

3x 15-second holds, 10-second rest between ➤

Pull-overs

10x ➤

Lunge Stretch + Knee Drop

2x 10-second holds, 7 knee drops, per side

Circuit Two—1x

Wide Founder with Tracing + Hold + Gorilla Reaches

- 7x Traces
- 10-second holds
- 10x Gorilla Reaches alternating arms ➤

Body Weight Squat

12x ➤

Woodpecker

- 15-second holds
- 10 hinges
- 10 rotations, per side

Core Round—1x

Janda Crunch

7x ➤

Oblique Roll

10x ➤

Eight-Point Plank Row

5x 2-second holds at the top, per side

Goblet Squat Hold—4.5 minutes

Cardio

30 minutes low-intensity. **Optional:** Go 10 minutes on 3 machines.

Recovery

Lat-to-Rotator Cuff Smash

2 minutes per side ➤

Pigeon Stretch

2 minutes per side

Activation—1x

Ankle Mobility	Bird Dogs	T-Spine Rotations	Glute Bridges	Goblet Squat	Behind the Back Hinge
10 pulses outward, middle and inward for each ankle ➤	10x alternating sides ➤	10x per side ➤	10x bridges, 10x extensions ➤	10x ➤	10x

Core Round—2x

Standing Plank with Band	Roll-outs on Stability Ball
7x extending straight up, 7x circles, per side ➤	Draw the alphabet A–Z

Circuit One—3x

Goblet Squat Walk	Pushup Walk	Romanian Dead Lifts + Hip Hinge Row
4x 3x Goblet Squat, walk 6 steps ➤	Got to 1 before failure ➤	8x per exercise

Circuit Two—3x

Getups	Kettlebell Swing	Farmer Carries
1x per side ➤	15x ➤	30-second walk

Cardio

Warm Up: 1 minute easy, 2x 30-seconds at 80% effort with 30 seconds off between sets.

Main Set: Tabata Cardio Workout
- **First Machine:** 8x 20-second sprints at 85–90% effort, 10 second rest
- 2 minutes recovery
- **Second Machine:** 8x 20-second sprints at 85–90% effort, 10 second rest

Cool Down: Go easy for two minutes

Recovery

Adductor Stretch	Calf Smash
2 minutes per side ➤	2 minutes per leg

Activation—1x

Ankle Mobility	Bird Dogs	T-Spine Rotations	Glute Bridges	Goblet Squat	Behind the Back Hinge
10 pulses outward, middle and inward for each ankle ➤	10x alternating sides ➤	10x per side ➤	10x bridges, 10x extensions ➤	10x ➤	10x

Core Round—2x

Eight-Point Plank Row	Janda Crunch
7x per side, alternating ➤	7x

Circuit One—2x

Bulgarian Split Squat	Pushups
2x • 5x right leg, 20-second rest • 5x left leg, 20-second rest ➤	4x 5 explosive, 30 seconds rest between

Circuit Two—5x

Kettlebell Swing	Pull-overs	Getups
15x ➤	10x ➤	1x per side

Cardio

Warm Up: 1 minute easy, 2x 30-seconds at 80% effort with 30 seconds off between sets.

Main Set:

• 6x 30-second sprint at 95+%, 90-second recovery between sprints

Cool Down: Go easy for two minutes

Recovery

Couch Stretch	T-Spine Smash
2 minutes per side ➤	4 minutes

MOVEMENT PRACTICE: Circuit One—1x

Founder

3x 15-second holds, 10-second rest between ➤

Pull-overs

10x ➤

Lunge Stretch + Knee Drop

2x 10-second holds, 7 knee drops, per side

Circuit Two—1x

Wide Founder with Tracing + Hold + Gorilla Reaches

- 7x Traces
- 10-second holds
- 10x Gorilla Reaches alternating arms ➤

Body Weight Squat

12x ➤

Woodpecker

- 10-second holds
- 10 hinges
- 10 rotations, per side

Core Round—5x

Getups

1 per side

Goblet Squat Hold—4.5 minutes

Cardio

30 minutes low-intensity. **Optional:** Go 10 minutes on 3 machines.

Recovery

Glute/TFL Smash

2 minutes per side ➤

Psoas Smash

2 minutes per side

Activation—1x

Ankle Mobility	Bird Dogs	T-Spine Rotations	Glute Bridges	Goblet Squat	Behind the Back Hinge
10 pulses outward, middle and inward for each ankle ➤	10x alternating sides ➤	10x per side ➤	10x bridges, 10x extensions ➤	10x ➤	10x

Core Round—2x

Eight-Point Plank Rows	Roll-outs on Stability Ball
7x per side, alternating ➤	Draw the alphabet A–Z

Circuit One—4x
(Take 30-second rests between each exercise, 2 minutes after each round.)

Goblet Squat Walk	Pushup Walk	Romanian Dead Lift + Hip Hinge Row	Farmer Carries
4x 3x Goblet Squat, walk 6 steps ➤	Go to 1 before failure ➤	7x per exercise ➤	Walk for 30 seconds

Cardio

Warm Up: 1 minute easy, 2x 30-seconds at 80% effort with 30 seconds off between sets.

Main Set: 2x

- 4x 15 Kettlebell Swings, 30-second rest between
- 1x 5 minutes at 85% effort, 2 minute rest between

Cool Down: Go easy for two minutes

Recovery

Pec Smash	Hamstring Smash
2 minutes per pec ➤	2 minutes per leg

Circuit One—1x

Founder

3x 15-second holds, 10-second rest between ➤

Pull-overs

10x ➤

Lunge Stretch + Knee Drop

2x 10-second holds, 10 knee drops, per side

Circuit Two—1x

Wide Founder with Tracing + Hold + Gorilla Reaches

- 7x Traces
- 10-second holds
- 10x Gorilla Reaches alternating arms ➤

Body Weight Squat

12x ➤

Woodpecker

- 10-second holds
- 10 hinges
- 10 rotations, per side

Core Round—1x

Eight-Point Plank Row

10x per side, alternating ➤

Weighted Side Plank

3x 10-second holds, per side ➤

Janda Crunch

7x

Goblet Squat Hold—5 minutes!

Cardio

30 minutes low-intensity.

Recovery

Diaphragm Smash

4 minutes ➤

Hamstring Stretch

2 minutes per side, contracting and releasing

STRENGTH MAINTENANCE: Activation—1x

Ankle Mobility	Bird Dogs	T-Spine Rotations	Glute Bridges	Goblet Squat	Behind the Back Hinge
10 pulses outward, middle and inward for each ankle ➤	10x alternating sides ➤	10x per side ➤	10x bridges, 10x extensions ➤	10x ➤	10x

Core Round—5x

Getups

1 per side

Circuit One—2x

Bulgarian Split Squat	Pushups
2x • 5x right leg, 20-second rest • 5x left leg, 20-second rest ➤	4x 5 explosive, 30 seconds rest between

Circuit Two—3x

Kettlebell Swing	Pull-overs	Getups
10x ➤	10x ➤	1x per side

Cardio

Warm Up: 1 minute easy, 2x 30-seconds at 80% effort with 30 seconds off between sets.

Main Set: 2x

• 4x 10-second sprints at 95% effort, 30-second recovery between sprints
• 2 minute rest between the two sets

Cool Down: Go easy for two minutes

Recovery

Lat-to-Rotator Cuff Roll	Pigeon Stretch
2 minutes per side ➤	2 minutes per side

Circuit One—1x

Founder

3x 15-second holds, 10-second rest between ➤

Pull-overs

10x ➤

Lunge Stretch + Knee Drop

2x 10-second holds, 10 knee drops, per side

Circuit Two—1x

Wide Founder with Tracing + Hold + Gorilla Reaches

- 7x Traces
- 10-second holds
- 10x Gorilla Reaches alternating arms ➤

Body Weight Squat

12x ➤

Woodpecker

- 10-second holds
- 10 hinges
- 10 rotations, per side

Circuit Three—1x

Eight-Point Plank Row

10x per side, alternating ➤

Roll-outs on Stability Ball

Draw the alphabet A–Z

Circuit Four—3x

Kettlebell Swing

4x 7 explosive swings, 30-second rest between ➤

Pushups

4x 5 pushups, 30-second rest between

Goblet Squat Hold—5 minutes

Recovery

Adductor Stretch

2 minutes per side ➤

Calf Smash

2 minutes per leg

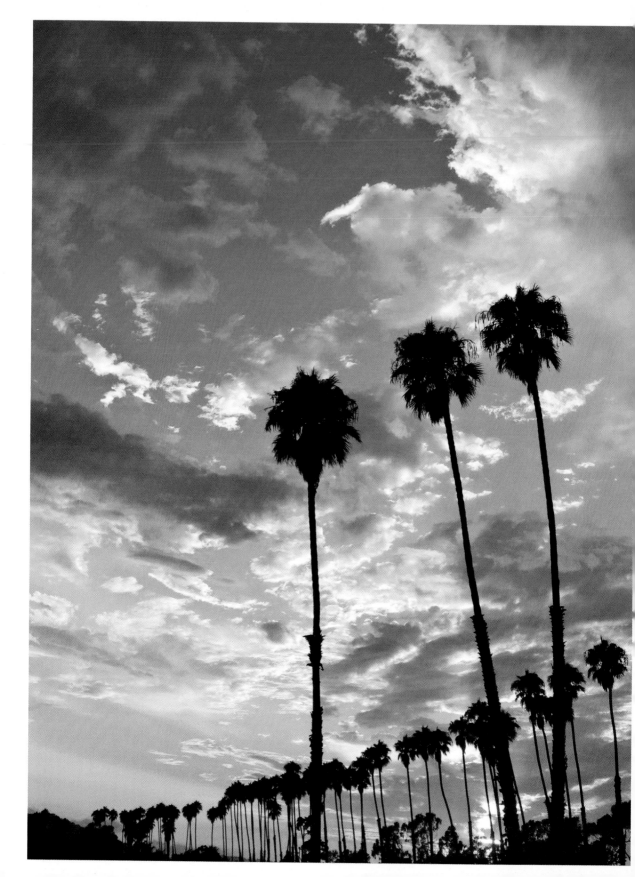

EPILOGUE

QUESTION: Okay, I switched my diet to one rich in healthy fats, I ditched almost all sugar and most carbs, and I made it through all the workouts (except Saturday Mornings—are you nuts?) I am fitter, no doubt, and the knee and lower back pain I had is pretty much gone. I even started running again for the first time in forever! But now what? Am I good to go? Am I rebounded for life? Can I stop training and start eating carbs and sugar again?

ANSWER: You can do anything you want. You decide your own fate. But if you stop training now, all the gains you've made will dry up like so much sweat, and all your effort and hard work will have been for naught.

You could go back through Rebound, starting with East Beach but changing things up. For instance, as you go through all the workouts again, try to keep laser focused on technique. Or increase your circuits to four times or five times through, cut down the number of reps, increase your weight, or try a new cardio machine you've successfully avoided so far.

If you don't want to keep doing the workouts in this book, you're likely now fit enough and have a high enough fitness IQ to try a new challenge. A lot of people get really hooked on CrossFit or training for a triathlon or a marathon. You could join a team that fits your skills and schedule, like a tennis group or a volleyball or basketball team. Or you could visit Pavel's website, strongfirst.com, and learn more about kettlebell training, a whole sport in and of itself. Don't limit yourself. Now's the time to break out and try something new.

That's what Rebounding is all about. Taking on new challenges, never getting stale, reinventing yourself over and over to become the strongest, most adaptable person you can be—just like my guinea pigs, John, Mike, and Chip. Thanks, guys! This book followed the stories of people I've worked with and for whom fitness has changed their lives. I hope it has helped you as well.

INDEX

couch stretch
  for ankles, 48
  example of, 46
  instructions for, 89, 89 (photo)
  for low back, 51
croissants, 15
CrossFit, 223

D

dairy, 14
dead lifts
  as basic exercise, 31, 37
  kettlebells, 155–157, 156–157 (photo)
  Romanian, 119, 119 (photo), 177–179,
    177–179 (photo)
  Romanian, with rows, 202, 202
    (photo)
desserts, 15
diabetes rates, 9
diaphragm smash
  importance of, 51
  with six-inch ball, 93, 93 (photo)
diets
  breakdown of, 13–15
  of Cappello, 6
  carb-loading types of, 4–5
  desserts in, 15
  difficulty in, 113–114
  failure of, 7
  of fats, 5–8
  frequent questions about, 7–11
  healthy ratios in, 10
  intuitive approach to, 10
  low-fat, 9
  Paleo, 8
  pasta in, 15
  shift in, 3–4, 6
  tips for, 66–67
  vegetables in, 3, 6, 7
dinner
  left overs from, 11–12

portion size during, 13–14
protein during, 13
donuts, 15
dumbbells
  bench press with, 39, 179–181,
    180–181 (photo)
  kettlebells versus, 39

E

East Beach
  new exercises for, 115–131, 115–131
    (photo)
  schedules for, 132–143
  starting out in, 113
  week four of, 141–143
  week one of, 132–134
  week three of, 138–140
  week two of, 135–137
eating
  disorders, 3
  habits, 3–4
eccentric movement, 59
eggs, 6, 13
eight-point plank, 72, 72 (photo)
  row, 238–239, 238–239 (photo)
  with reach-out, 182–183, 182–183
    (photo)
elliptical machine, 25
endurance athlete
  calories of, 4
  energy of, 5
energy
  aerobic, 5
  of endurance athlete, 5
  gels, 5
  during Ironman triathlon, 4–5
  sugar for, 4

F

farmer carries
  in circuit training, 39